JOHN TRAVOLTA

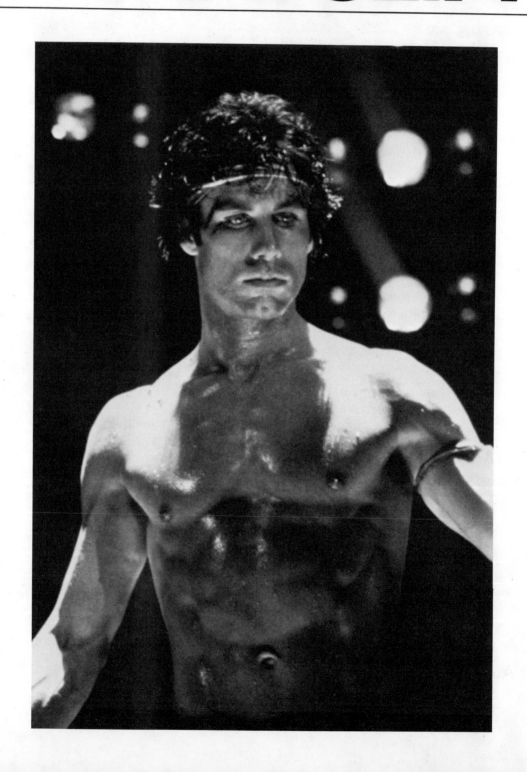

STAYING FIT!

His complete program
for reshaping
your body through
weight resistance training
and modern dance techniques

Weight Training Program designed with
Dan Isaacson

Dance Exercise Program designed with
Dennon and Sayhber Rawles

SIMON AND SCHUSTER

NEW YORK

Note to the Reader

This book is designed to set forth the exercise, diet, and other regimes which I have successfully followed, but my programs are not intended to be undertaken without the reader's initially and regularly checking with his or her doctor or health care professional.

Published by Simon and Schuster
A Division of Simon & Schuster, Inc.
Simon & Schuster Building
Rockefeller Center
1230 Avenue of the Americas
New York, New York 10020
SIMON AND SCHUSTER and colophon are registered trademarks
of Simon & Schuster, Inc.

Manufactured in the United States of America

10 9 8 7 6 5 4 3 2 1

Library of Congress Cataloging in Publication Data

Travolta, John, date.
John Travolta's Creative exercising.

1. Exercise. 2. Dancing. 3. Weight
lifting. 4. Hygiene. I. Title. II. Title:
Creative exercising.
GV481.T67 1984   613.7'1   84-5506
ISBN 0-671-49798-7

The author gratefully acknowledges
permission to reproduce photographs from
Paramount Pictures.

Exercise photographs by Jim Fridley
Photographs of Dan Isaacon by John Balik
Hairstyle by Rico

Acknowledgments

I would like to thank the following people for keeping me in good shape:

☐ Marilu Henner, my partner in the couples exercises,

☐ Sly for showing me the way and changing my life,

☐ Dan Isaacson for his expertise in training and all his love and support,

☐ Sharee Lane for literally changing me into a professional dancer,

☐ Dennon and Sayhber Rawles for giving me choreography that put my efforts into high form,

☐ Fred Gaines, for all his good advice

☐ John Herman for his editorial help,

☐ Marcelle Baldo for keeping my hair and scalp in such good condition,

☐ Margie Luiza for keeping my face and skin so healthy,

☐ Dr. An Than for his brilliant work in the field of herbal medicine,

☐ The Universal and Paramount Equipment Companies for providing the machines that helped me make my goals come to fruition,

☐ Randy Eighmy and Bob Hamlin for use of their weight training and dance facilities for the photo sessions in the book,

☐ Dennis Tinerino, Mr. Universe, technical consultant and professional body builder for his assistance during the photo session,

☐ And last but not least, the people at Sundance in Encino, California, for providing the Sontegra Tanning Machine that added the golden touch.

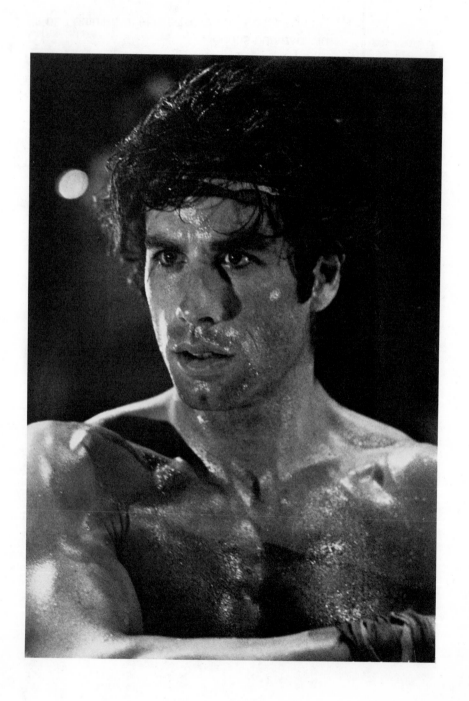

Contents

PREFACE 9

STAYING FIT! 11

WARM-UP 15

DANCE EXERCISES 17

ISOLATION / 19

STANDING STRETCH / 34
BEGINNERS / 34
INTERMEDIATE / 47
ADVANCED / 52

FLOOR STRETCH / 58
BEGINNERS / 58
INTERMEDIATE / 80
ADVANCED / 88

STANDING STRETCH FINISH / 98
BEGINNERS / 98
INTERMEDIATE / 109
ADVANCED / 110

PARTNER STRETCH / 114

COOL-DOWN / 136

MUSCLE CHART / 144-145

WEIGHT TRAINING 146

BEGINNERS / 149

INTERMEDIATE / 172

ADVANCED / 206

TIPS ON DIET AND HEALTH 249

DIET / 249

HAIR AND SKIN CARE / 251

STAYING IN SHAPE / 252

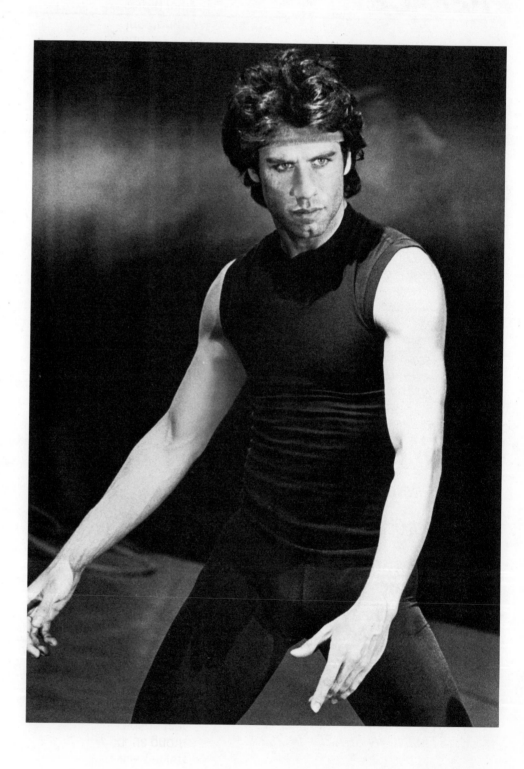

PREFACE

In order to play professional dancer Tony Manero in *Staying Alive*, I needed a lean muscular body with strong supple lines. I had four months to get into the best shape of my life. This was a terrific challenge—because I was in the worst shape of my life. I was twenty pounds overweight and I hadn't done any regular exercise for almost a year. If I was to reach my goal, I would need to work out full time—and I did! I worked six days a week for a minimum of five hours a day—and sometimes for fourteen hours a day!—throughout the entire rehearsal and shooting of the film. By the end I hardly recognized myself. I had really developed the strong lithe body I wanted.

That experience taught me incredible things about the body and what it can do—how it can be reshaped so you can make yourself over entirely, creating an entirely new you. I now look at bodies almost like pieces of clay that can be molded. All the potential is there, and great results can be achieved if you are willing to work at it, and if you have someone to show you the way.

That's why I'm writing this book. Of course my regime for *Staying Alive* was almost too much for anyone. Unless you are under the gun the way I was—and in my case a movie studio was pouring money into a new picture—you should give yourself a break and set a less intense rate of progress. But with the right program you can redesign your body—as I did, and as this book will show you how to do, too.

I know how much a personal trainer can mean, since I was lucky enough to have not only my own, Dan Isaacson, but also Sylvester Stallone watching over me to make sure that everything was going according to plan. That's why in this book I offer a personalized program with step-by-step instructions that provide the kind of one-on-one attention I had. As you can see from the pictures, this program worked for me.

My program features a regime of weight resistance training for the upper body, along with my own specially designed routine of dance exercises worked out with choreographers Dennon and Sayhber Rawles for developing aerobic capacity and strengthening the lower body. Combined with a strict protein diet, this was the program I used to get into shape for *Staying Alive*—with fantastic results!

It wouldn't be accurate if I didn't admit to cheating a little on the diet. Try to behave yourself—but it's even more important for the program to be right for you. As long as you are willing to work hard at the dance and weight-training exercises you can always make up for a minor slip in eating.

Believe me, it was difficult when I started my program to reshape my body, and it was difficult sometimes to see it through to the end—but it was definitely worth it! Now it's your turn. I think you're going to enjoy it. Soon it will be less work and a lot more fun—and the results can be terrific!

Good luck!

STAYING FIT!

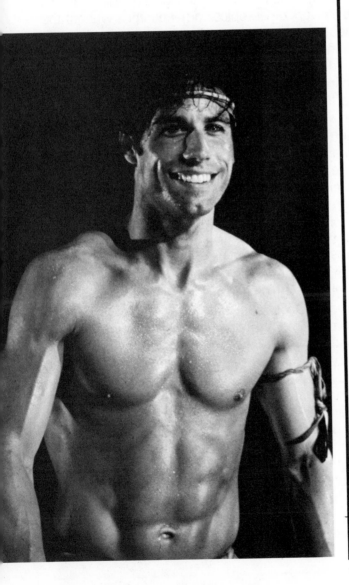

My book is designed to provide a six-day-a-week workout program combining the spontaneity and excitement of dance exercise with the building and toning of weight lifting. The program is divided into three parts—*warm-up,* which is to be done every day, and is closely integrated with the dance exercises; *dance exercises*—The Standing Stretch, Floor Stretch, Standing Stretch Finish, Partner Stretch (optional), and Cool-Down—to be performed every other day of the six-day cycle; and *weight training,* to be performed on the alternate days of the six-day cycle. Thus if you did the dance exercises on Monday, Wednesday, and Friday, you would do the weight training on Tuesday, Thursday, and Saturday. And on the seventh day you rest.

The six-day-a-week program can also be condensed into a three-day-a-week program by combining the dance and weight training on the same day. If you decide to do the three-day program, the dance exercises should precede the weight training. When you exercise in this way, you should exercise on every other day of the six-day cycle, and rest on the alternate days. Thus, if you exercised on Monday, Wednesday, and Friday, you would rest on Tuesday, Thursday, and Saturday.

You may not be able to do every exercise at first, but don't get discouraged. Your body will respond to repetition and consistency, and slowly as the weeks go by, you'll get there. I know. I was where you are now. So don't quit!

Taking up exercising is a little like learning to fly. When taking flying lessons, many people quit after the ninth or tenth hour of instruction. It's so hard and discouraging, they don't see any future. But if they'd just go on for another two hours, it would click. I quit flying at this point twice before I finally stuck with it and got it; and now flying is one of my favorite things.

The first few weeks of exercising are crucial—especially for the weight training program. The dancing is something different, at least for me—I'll get to that in a minute. But the weight training was murder. I was a *brat*—I admit it. If there was a way to put off the session, I tried. But somewhere around the fifth week something strange happened. Suddenly I had turned a corner—I *wanted* to work out. It was becoming addictive!

It's sort of like climbing a steep hill—it takes

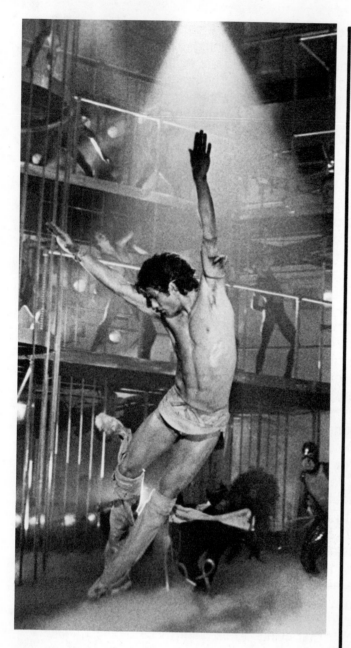

some puffing to get to the top, but once you're there it's easy going, and the view can be magnificent. Now if I skip a few days of exercise, I feel terrible. I look *forward* to it, and I can actually say I feel better at thirty than I did at twenty. I almost feel as if I have started all over!

Now let me say a little about the dance exercises. Dancing is what I enjoy most, and what I think is really exciting and new is combining dancing with weight training in a single, balanced program.

Any workout program needs to combine a number of elements if it is to be complete: Exercises to develop stretch and flexibility; aerobic exercises for endurance; and exercises for strength and muscular development. My program contains all these, but the really creative part is the dance, which allows you to work on aerobics and endurance without the monotony, or even boredom, of skipping rope or running in place or jogging or swimming laps. The dance music adds interest and excitement, and I've also included a section of exercises to be done with a partner. Working out with a friend is always better than working alone—especially when your partner is someone of the opposite sex!

Staying on a diet was really tough for me because I love to eat. At first my attitude toward diet and exercise was really hesitant, so believe me, I know where you're coming from. But with the help of Sly Stallone and Dan Isaacson I was able to keep on the diet, though at first it was hard. Often they ate with me to make sure I didn't cheat. Little did they know that sometimes I would stay up all night just imagining what it would be like to have another meal in my stomach. Occasionally I'd have to sneak a piece of fruit or some protein just to tide me over until breakfast. Some nights, especially early on, I found it very difficult to sleep because my body was used to having more food and less exercise. Now I was working out and eating less—it didn't seem fair! I remember having daydreams of burying my face in a whole chocolate cake and eating my way through it until I was finished! But I resisted. Then after about five weeks I began to see a huge difference in my body. Others had told me of the changes they saw before that—which is why weekly photos are a good idea as a way to keep track of your progress. Anyway, as I started to see my body getting into better shape, my appetite for food decreased—but my appetite for sex increased! Fortunately sex is not fattening, so treat yourself to it. It's even more fun when you're in good shape because you're proud of the way you look and feel.

Remember, once you're in shape it's not difficult to maintain, it's just getting there that's the real drag—and I mean drag. There's no way of getting around it. That's why it helps to have a partner or a trainer to keep you going when the going gets tough.

But one day soon, you'll look in the mirror and, wow! You won't believe the difference. After that it will be easy—so stick with it.

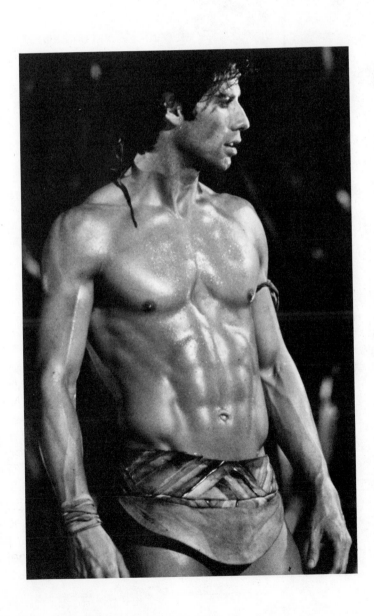

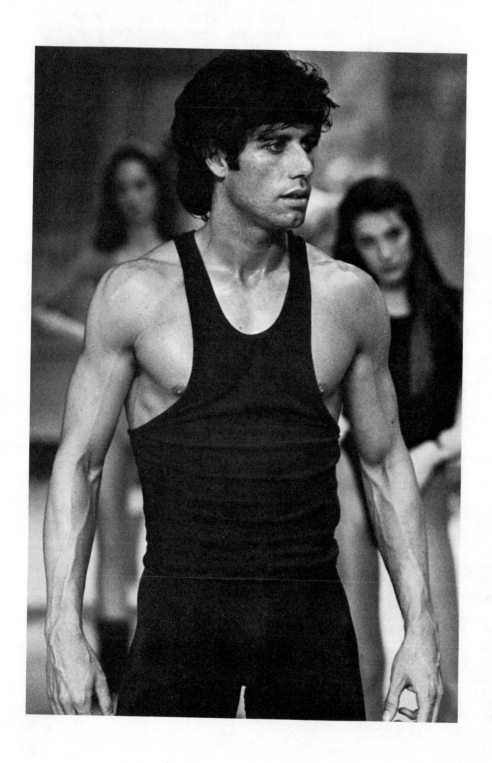

WARM-UP

It's essential you do some sort of warm-up before you get into the more strenuous part of any exercise program. This is so your muscles and joints get limbered and stretched and you don't strain or tear anything. Dancers always spend time warming up as a part of their regular routine. That's why in this book I've built the warm-up into the dance routine. The purpose of the Isolation exercises is not only to develop timing and coordination, but to loosen and warm up major muscle and joint areas in preparation for the other exercises. These exercises also help you develop an awareness and control of each of the various areas of your body.

Here then are the warm-up exercises I recommend for each session, depending on the exercise program you plan for that day: On the days you are doing only *Dance,* the warm-ups consist of the Isolation exercises. The workout consists of The Standing Stretch, Floor Stretch, Standing Stretch Finish, and Cool-down.

On the days you are doing only *Weight Training,* the warm-ups consists of all the Isolation exercises, plus the first seven exercises from the Beginners Standing Stretch (pages 34 through 45). These exercises are to be done consecutively, as given in the text.

On the days you are going both *Dance* and *Weight Training,* the warm-up consists of the Isolation exercises.

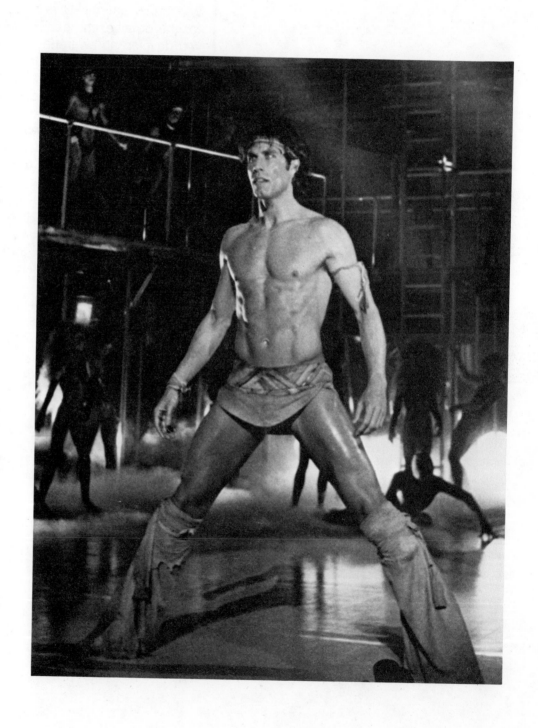

DANCE EXERCISES

Equipment needed for the dance exercises:

Clothing: One of the great things about the dance exercises is that you can do them wearing whatever is comfortable. You can wear a sweat outfit, or shorts and a T-shirt. If you like you can purchase dance clothing, which can be bought at any local dance-wear boutique. You can wear lightweight tennis shoes or go barefoot.

Music: Any of your favorite upbeat music that keeps a steady tempo is appropriate. You can use either cassettes or records, or you can turn on the radio to a station that plays music you like.

Towel: Keep a towel handy to wipe your face so the perspiration won't get into your eyes.

Mirror: If you have a large mirror to place in front of you, it can help you place your body in the correct positions.

Chair: For a number of the dance exercises you will need a chair with a high back to hold on to for balance.

Mats: You may want to purchase a floor mat to use for the floor exercises. However, a soft carpet will do just as well.

Isolation

APPROXIMATELY FOUR MINUTES FOR BEGINNERS, INTERMEDIATE AND ADVANCED. START YOUR MUSIC BEFORE BEGINNING.

The approximate times given are only a suggestion. They will vary depending upon the tempo of the music, your familiarity with the exercises, and your physical condition. Don't hesitate to add a few seconds between exercises to catch your breath, especially when you are just beginning the program.

Neck

The neck isolation exercises will increase the mobility in your neck muscles and the blood flow to your head.

Starting Position: Stand with your legs approximately two feet apart and your feet in a parallel position, with toes pointing forward. Place your hands on your hips with elbows out to the side. Stand up straight, keep your stomach muscles lifted up, and relax your shoulders.

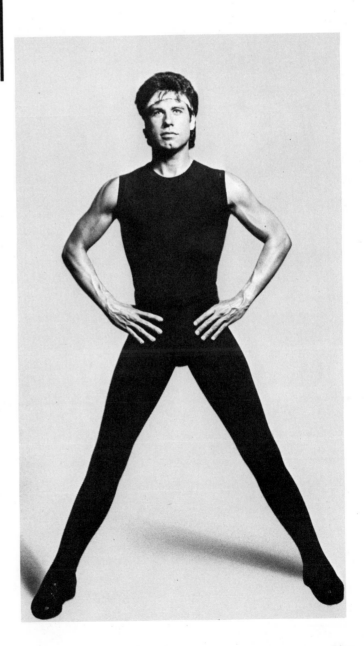

SIDE TO SIDE

Description: Place your right ear down toward your right shoulder, then swing your head up and over so your left ear is down toward your left shoulder.

Repetitions: Using 2 counts to go to each side, bring your ear to your shoulder four times on each side. Then do a faster 1-count on each side for a total of eight repetitions on each side.

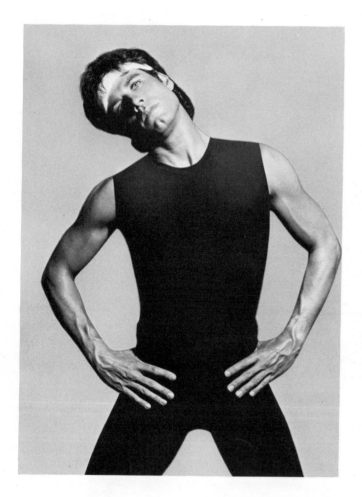 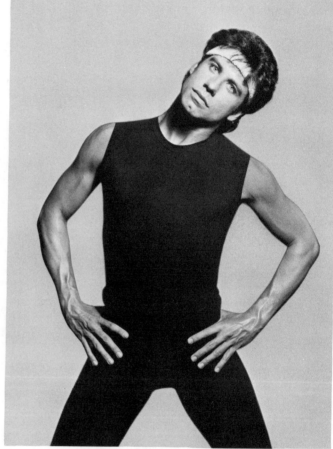

FORWARD AND BACK

Description: Drop your head forward, placing your chin on your chest. Then lift your head up and back as far as you can until you are looking straight up, or even farther back, without lifting your shoulders.

Repetitions: Use the same counts as for the Side to Side isolation.

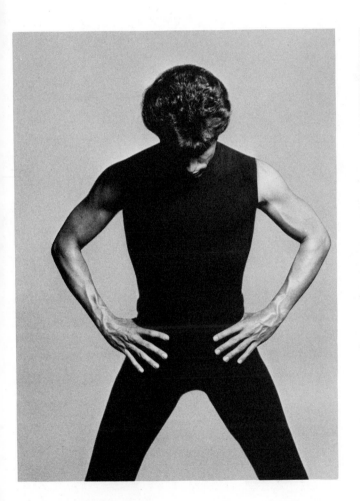
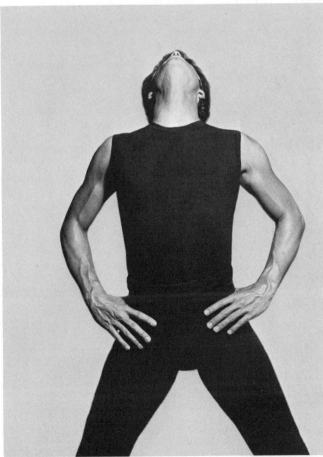

SPOTTING RIGHT AND LEFT

Description: Turn your head to look over your right shoulder without moving your upper body or lifting your shoulder, then pass through your starting position and look over your left shoulder.

Repetitions: Again use the same counts and number of repetitions as for the Side to Side.

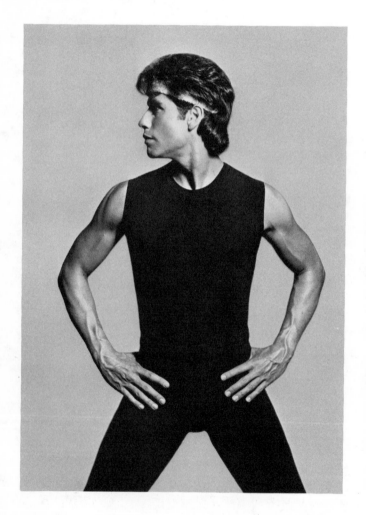
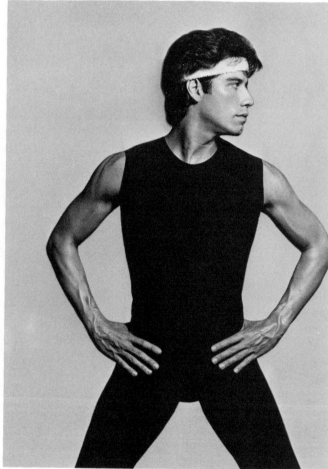

CIRCLING

Description: Half circle: Start by placing your right ear over to the right shoulder. Roll your head down through the position where your chin is on your chest, then up to the position where the left ear is on the left shoulder. Then reverse the movement.

Full circle: Start by doing the half circle from right ear to left, then continue rolling your head without stopping until the chin is up, and you are looking up. Continue around to the right ear and finish with your head down and chin on your chest.

Repetitions: Use 4 counts to complete one half-circle movement, right to left, and 4 counts to reverse, going from left to right. Do a total of four repetitions on each side. Then without stopping continue to the full circle, using 8 counts to complete one circle right around to chin on chest, and then 8 counts to reverse the direction. Do a total of four repetitions in each direction, alternating direction.

Note: *In the intermediate and advanced programs, the above circling isolation can be done using 2 counts for the half circle and 4 counts for the whole circle.*

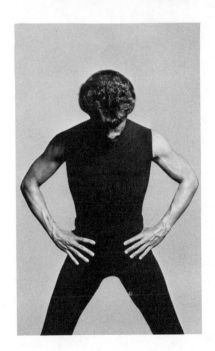
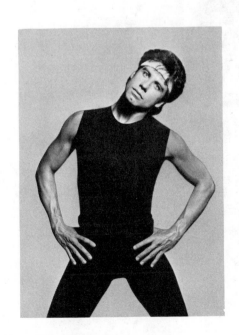
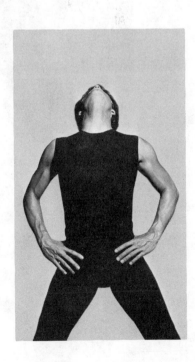

Shoulders

Great for easing tension in your neck and shoulders.

Starting position: Keep your legs apart about two feet, and place your arms down by your sides. Keep your elbows locked straight, palms facing forward, fingers stretched.

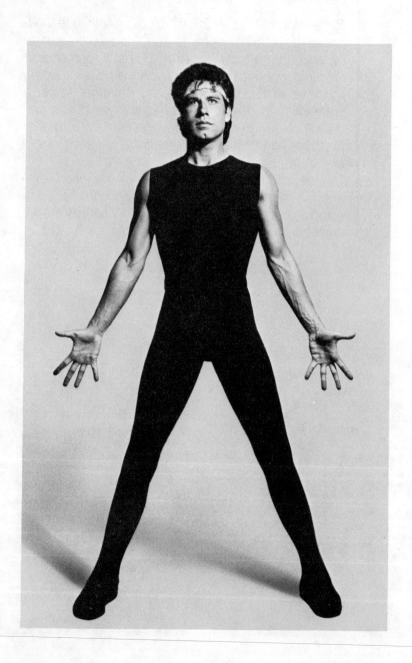

UP AND DOWN

Description: Raise your shoulders to your ears in a shrug position and release them down to a relaxed position.

Repetitions: Use 2 counts to take shoulders up to your ears and 2 counts to lower them. Do this a total of four times. Then increase the speed to 1 count up and 1 count down for a total of eight repetitions.

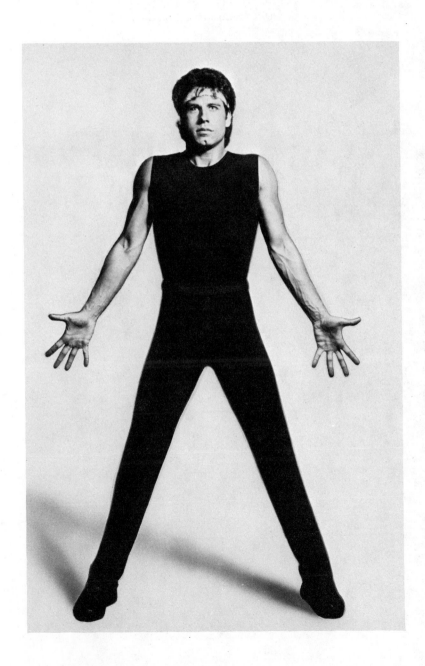

CIRCLING

Description: Start by bringing your shoulders forward and raising them to your ears, then pull them back by pulling your shoulder blades together. Relax them down. Then reverse the circle by starting back and up, then pushing your shoulders forward and releasing them down.

Repetitions: Use 4 counts for each circle. Do four consecutive circles up and back around, then four consecutive circles going up and forward. Then increase speed, using only 2 counts for each circle. Do four circles back and four circles front.

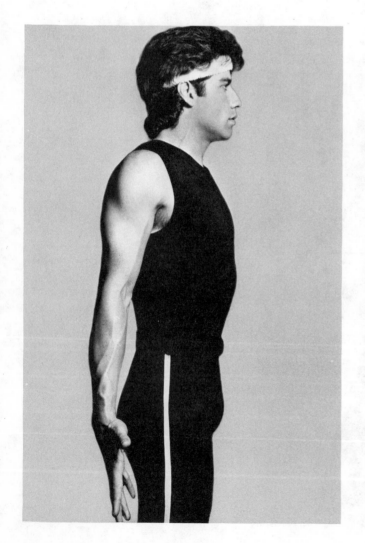
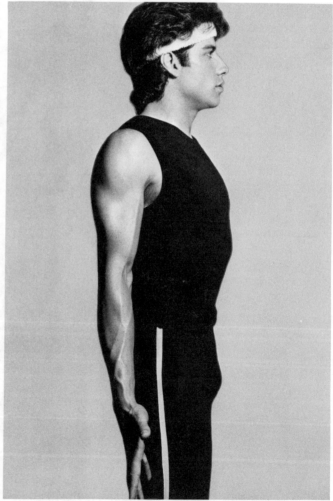

Rib cage

Great for your spine and sides.

Starting position: *Keep the same leg position as in the shoulder exercises. Extend your arms straight out to the side from your shoulders, palms facing forward, fingers stretched.*

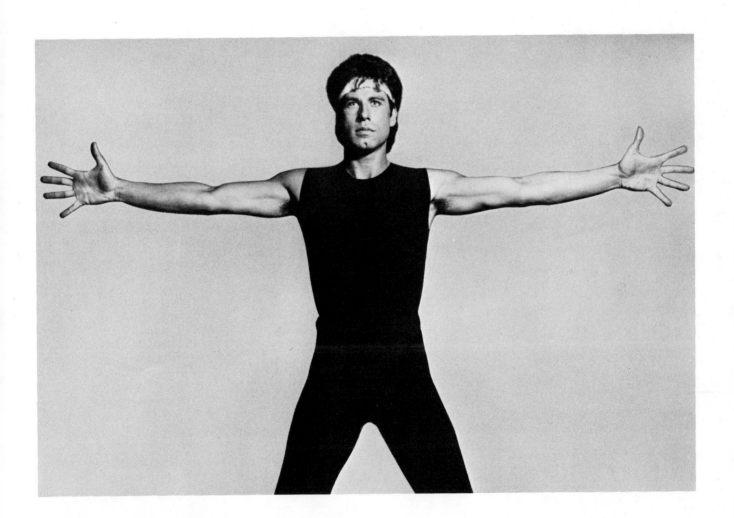

SIDE TO SIDE

Description: You want to feel as if you are reaching your entire torso over to the side. Allow your body from your waist up to move over to the right. Then move your torso over to the left. Keep your arms still, your hips immobile, and your shoulders relaxed.

Repetitions: Use 2 counts to reach to the right, and 2 counts to reach to the left. Do a total of four on each side, then increase speed to 1 count on each side, for a total of eight on each side.

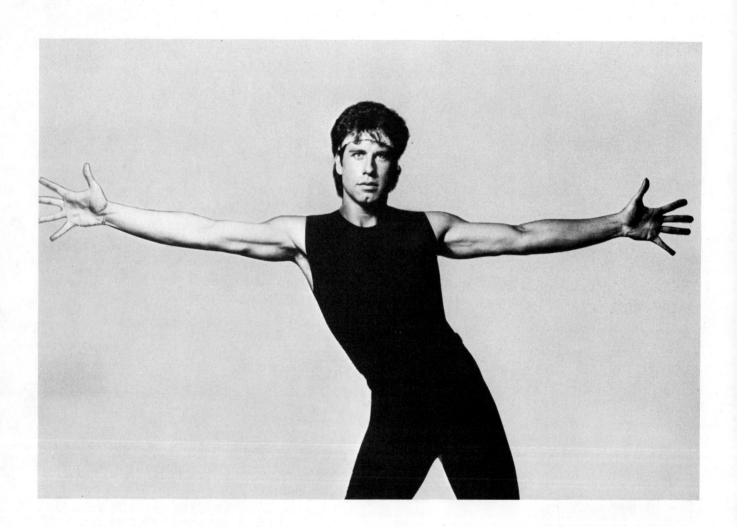

FRONT TO BACK

Description: Place your hands on your hips. Begin by pushing your chest forward, making your back arch. Then move your chest back, and contract your rib cage to a concave, rounded position. Remember to keep your hips immobile.

Repetitions: Use 2 counts to push forward and arch, and 2 counts to contract and round. Do a total of four repetitions in each direction. Then increase speed to 1 count forward and 1 count back. Do eight more repetitions in each direction.

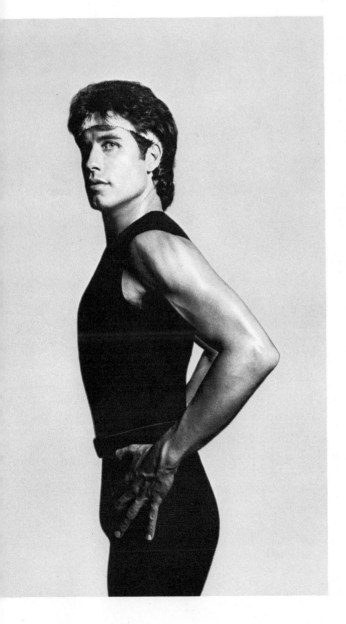

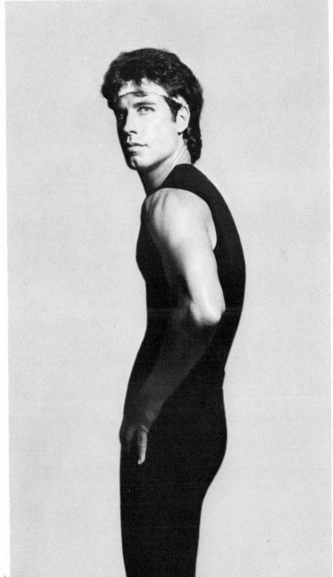

Hips

Great for the hip joints and for tightening the buttocks.

Starting position: Stand with your legs apart, toes pointing forward. Now bend your knees and relax your arms at your sides.

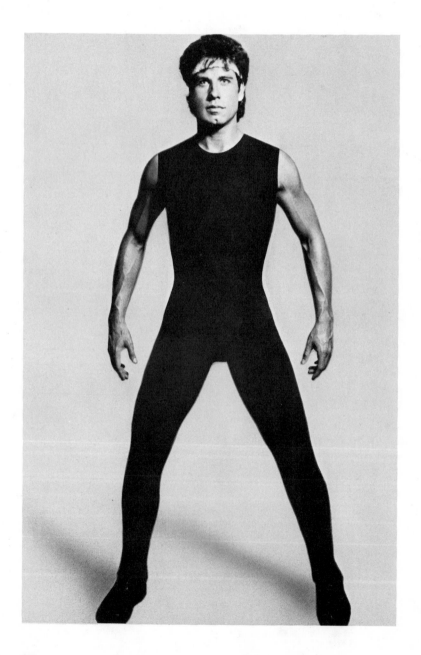

SIDE TO SIDE

Description: Shift your hip to the right side until you feel your weight resting on your right hip. Then repeat the same on the left side. Keep your feet flat and immobile on the floor.

Repetitions: Use 2 counts in each direction. Do a total of four repetitions on each side. Then increase speed to 1 count and do eight more repetitions.

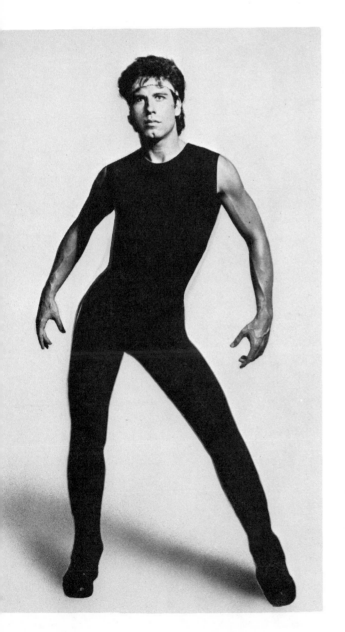 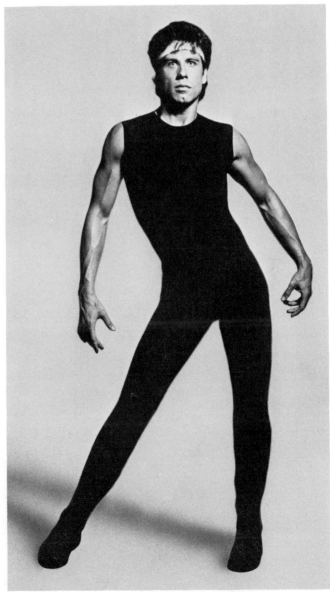

FRONT AND BACK

Description: Thrust your hips forward and tighten your buttocks. Then release your hips back, sticking your buttocks out in an arched position. Work to keep your rib cage still.

Repetitions: Use 2 counts in each direction. Do a total of four repetitions in each direction. Then increase speed to 1 count and do eight more repetitions in each direction.

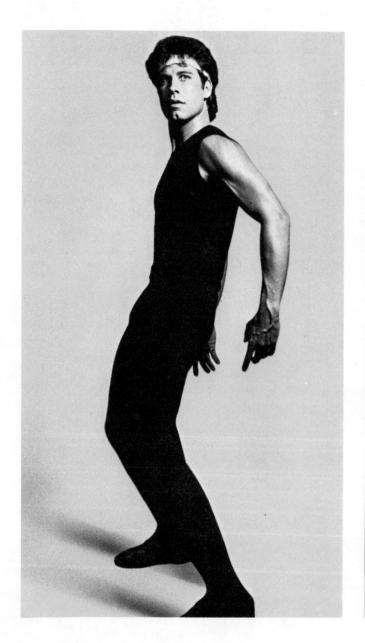
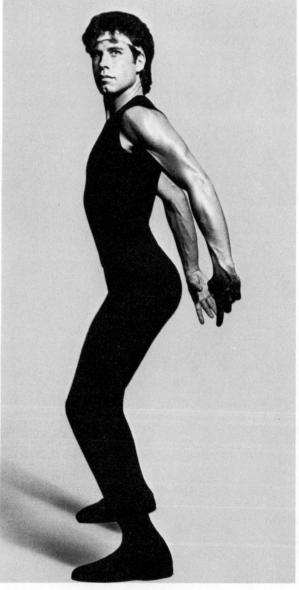

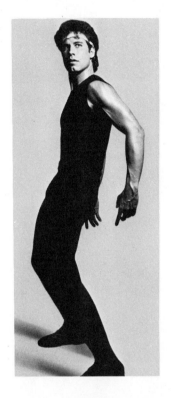

CIRCLING

Description: Keep your knees bent and start the circle by pushing your hips forward. Swing them to the right side, then to the back-arch position, around to the left, then front.

Repetitions: Use 4 counts for each circle. Do four continuous circles going front-right-back-left, and then four continuous circles going front-left-back-right-around. Then increase speed, using only 2 counts per circle. Do eight repetitions in 2 counts.

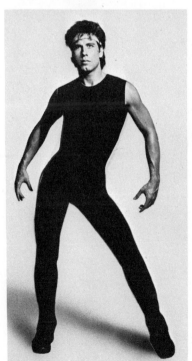

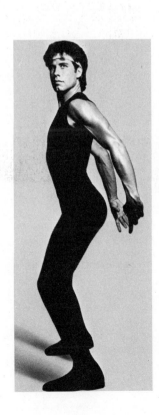

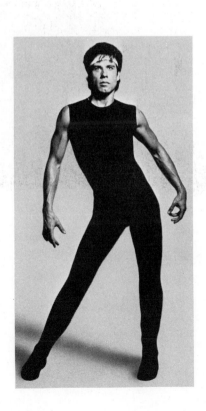

Standing Stretch

BEGINNERS
APPROXIMATELY SIX MINUTES

Starting position: Stand with your legs straight and opened about two feet apart. Place your feet in a parallel position pointing straight forward. Extend both arms over your head, straight up from your shoulders.

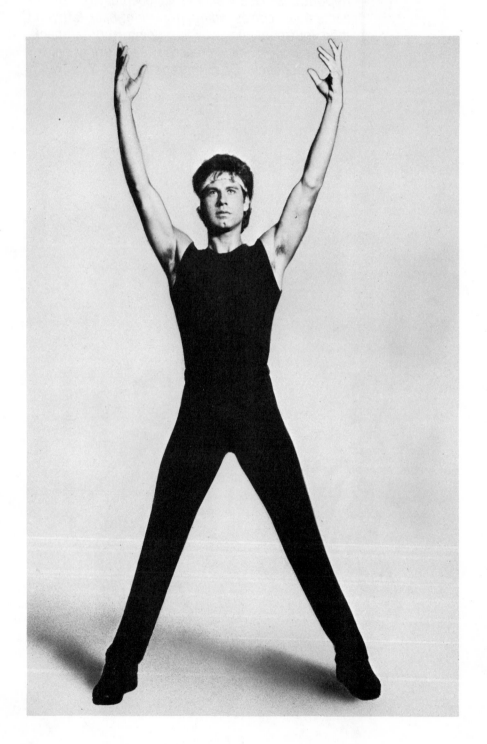

REACHING STRETCH

Description: Reach up alternating arms, using first your right arm, then your left. The feeling is that of trying to touch or grab something just a few inches out of your reach.

Repetitions: Take 2 counts for each Arm Reach and do a total of four repetitions on each side. Then increase your speed so that each reach is done in 1 count.

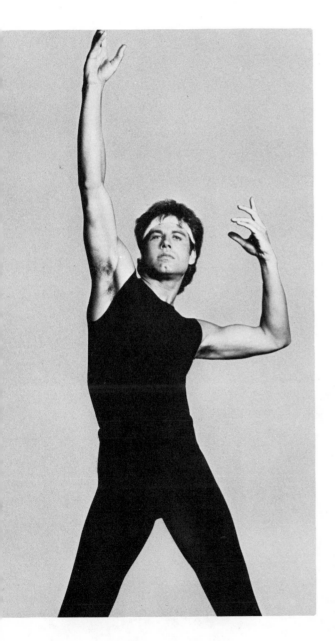

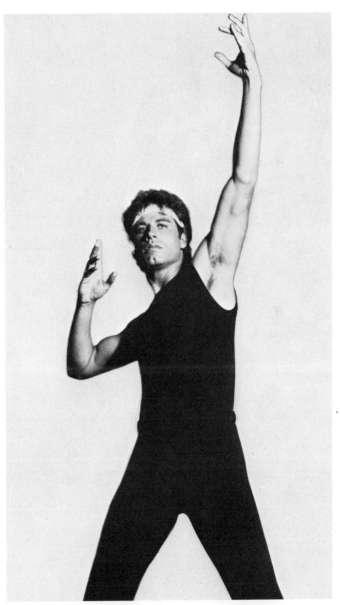

ARCH-DOWN AND ROLL-UP

Description: The Arch-Down is done by bending your knees and slowly lowering your arms to your sides. You need to look up as you descend and allow your hips to release back so your back becomes completely arched. The Roll-Up is the opposite of the arch: At the bottom of the arched position, let your head drop and your back round, so you are now looking at the floor. Begin to straighten your legs slowly and keep your chin to your chest until your legs are completely straight, then lift your chin so you are back in the starting position.

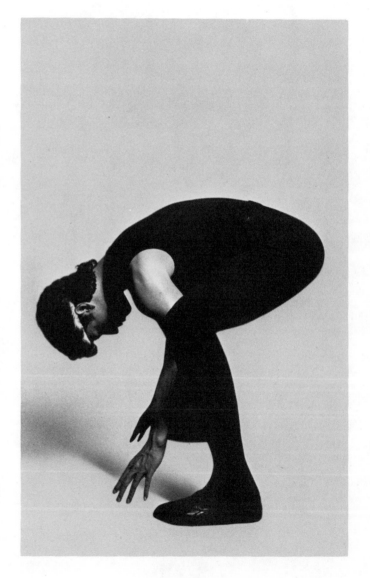

Repetitions: Take 8 counts to arch down and 8 counts to roll up. Do this sequence twice. Then increase the speed so the Arch-Down is done in 4 counts, and the Roll-Up in 4 counts. Do this sequence twice.

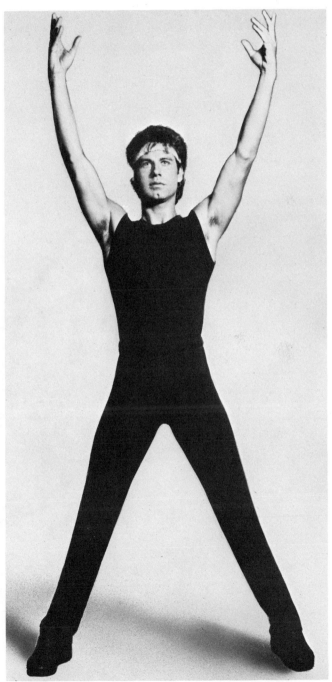

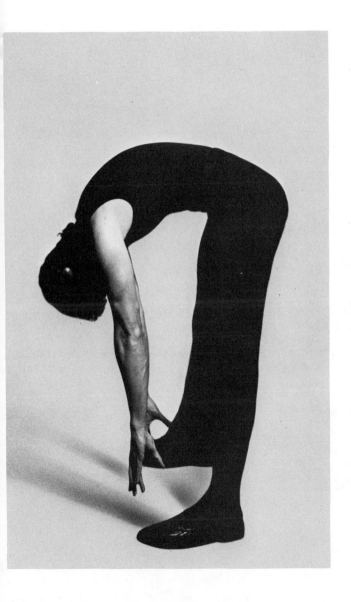

SIDE STRETCH

Description: Start with both hands on your hips. Then bend over sideways to the right and bring your left arm over your head. The feeling is that of reaching over to the right wall. Change arms and bend to the left with your right arm over your head, reaching for the left wall.

Repetitions: Take 8 counts, using a slight bounce on each count, to stretch to the right, and 8 counts to stretch to the left. Repeat. Then increase the speed by using only 4 counts on each side. Repeat.

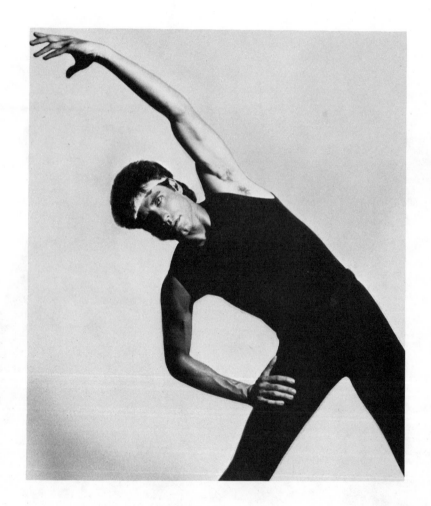

FORWARD STRETCH AND HIP PUSH

Description: Keeping your legs straight with your feet still parallel, start by bending forward from the waist. Reach your arms out to the side and keep your back in a straight, flat line. Do easy bounces in this position.

Then straighten up, place your hands on the back of your hips, and in a rocking motion push your hips forward, doing easy bounces.

Repetitions: Do eight bounces forward and eight bounces pushing the hips. Do twice in 8 counts and then twice in 4 counts.

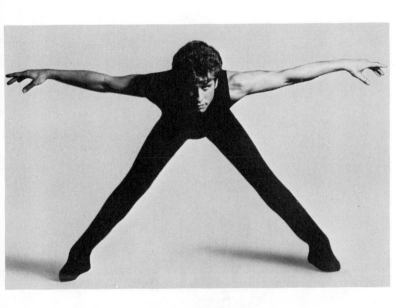

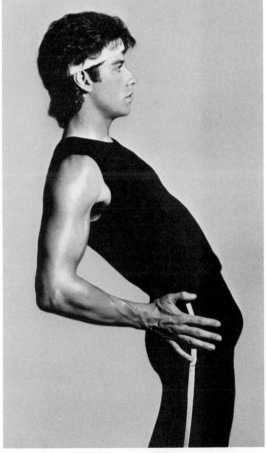

LEG LUNGES

Description: Keep your legs apart as before, but now turn your feet out to the side. Place your hands on your hips. You will begin by bending your right knee. Keep your right knee directly in line with your right toes. Keep your back straight, your stomach lifted, and keep your right heel on the floor when you are bending.

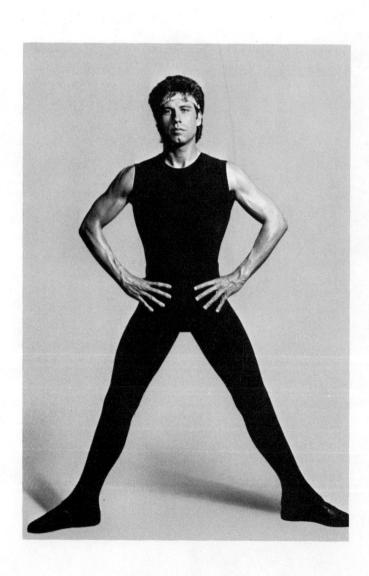

Repetitions: *Take 4 counts to bend your right knee and 4 counts to straighten it. Then do the same with your left leg. Repeat. Then use only 2 counts going down and 2 counts coming up. Do this twice.*

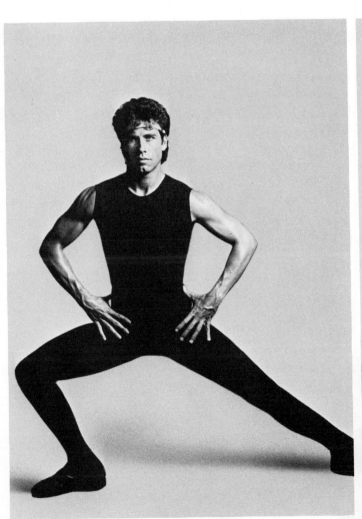

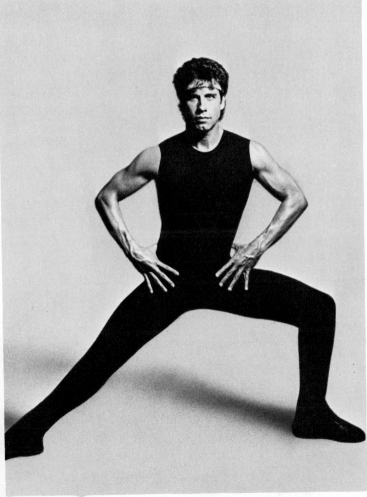

PLIÉS IN SECOND POSITION AND HEEL LIFTS

The Pliés will work the tops of your thighs, and the Heel Lifts will tighten and develop your calves.

Description: Keeping your legs apart and your feet turned out ("second position"), bend both legs at the same time. Keep your knees in line with your toes as you descend slowly halfway to the floor. Then bounce in place, and slowly come up to the starting position.

The heel lifts are done while you are in the plié (bent-knee) position—your heels on the floor and your knees pointing out over your toes. Lift one heel at a time as high as you can, keeping your weight evenly distributed between both legs. When you lift

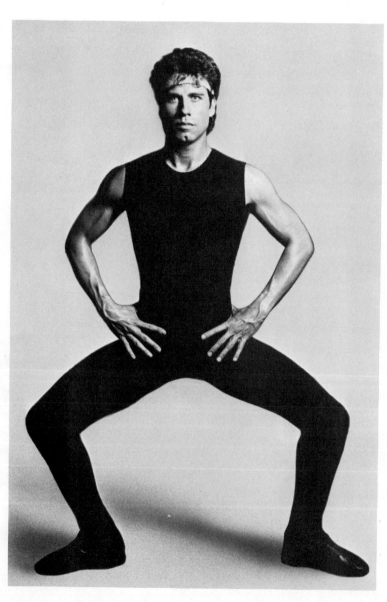

the heel, your weight will be on the ball of your foot. Do easy bounces in this position. Then release the heel back down and repeat, using the other foot.

Repetitions: Take 4 counts to descend into the plié. Do four bounces in place and take 4 counts to ascend to the starting position. Do this twice in 4 counts and then twice in 2 counts.

Return to the plié and hold for 8 counts before beginning the heel lifts. Then lift your right heel off the floor and do four bounces, lower that heel and lift the left heel for four bounces. Repeat on each leg.

Now stand up, relax and shake your legs and arms a bit. This will relieve any unwanted tension in your body.

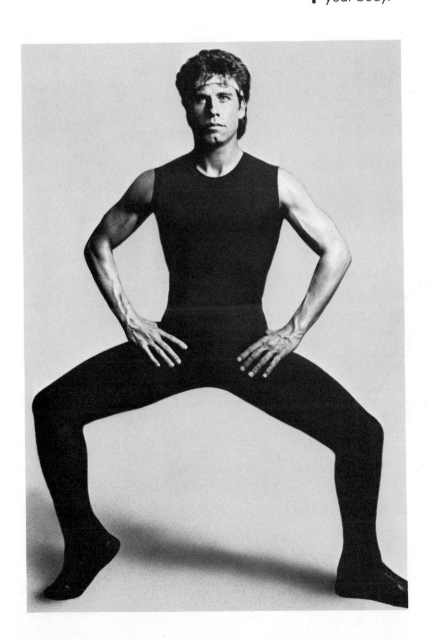

STRETCH AND SQUAT

Description: Start with legs apart, toes pointed forward in a parallel position. Begin by bending over at the waist to allow your head to be as close to the floor as possible. Take hold of your ankles or calves and give a gentle pull as if trying to get your head through your legs.

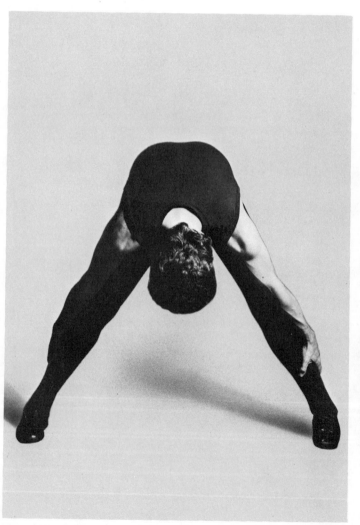
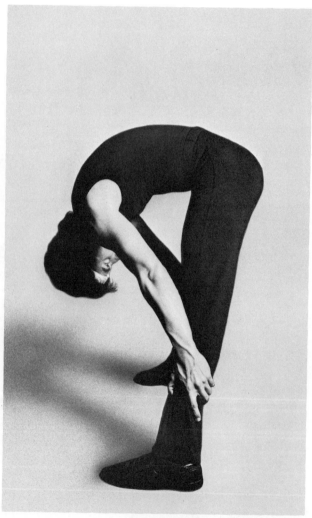

Then, while still holding on to your ankles, bend your knees and squat. Your knees should be pointing forward, and you should look straight forward.

Repetitions: Use 8 counts to stretch forward, holding on to your ankles. Then 8 counts in the squat position doing a bounce on each count. Do this twice in 8 counts and twice in 4 counts.

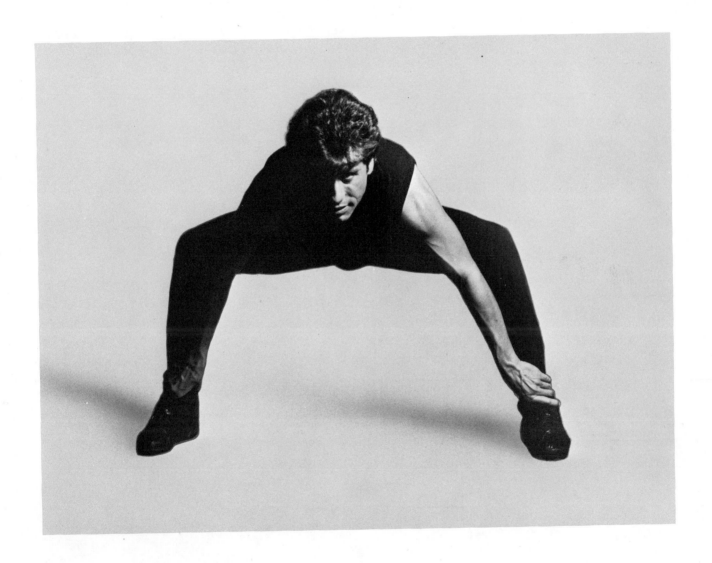

The following is a transition exercise to take you from the Stretch and Squat to the floor exercises.

OPEN SIDE SPLIT

Description: From an upright position, keeping your legs straight and your feet parallel, bend over from the waist and place your palms on the floor. If this is difficult, open your legs a few inches wider until this can be accomplished. Support your weight with your arms and slowly slide your legs open as far as you can. Do not overdo this at first. Just slide your legs until you feel your inner leg muscles stretching.

Repetitions: Slide your legs into the Open Slide Split and hold for 8 counts. Then slowly ease yourself down onto the floor in a sitting position.

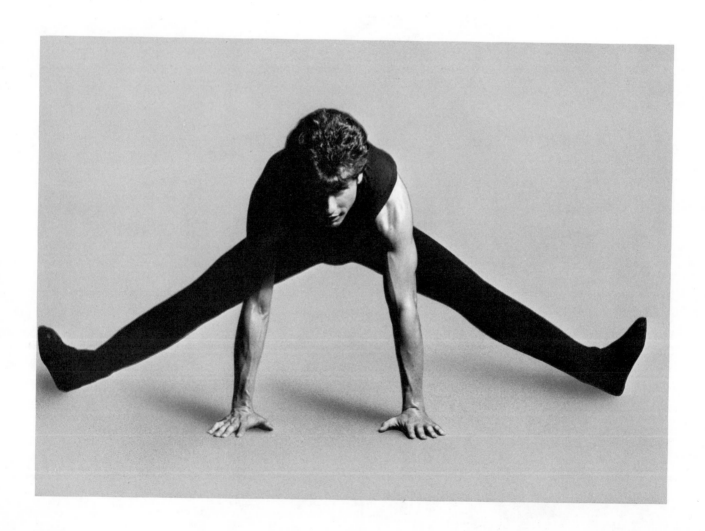

Standing Stretch

INTERMEDIATE
APPROXIMATELY SEVEN MINUTES

REACHING STRETCH

Do the exercise as described in the beginners Standing Stretch (page 35).

ARCH-DOWN AND ROLL-UP

Do the exercise as described in the beginners Standing Stretch (page 36).

SIDE STRETCH

Do the beginners version first (page 38), then repeat in 2 counts twice, then 1 count twice.

FORWARD STRETCH AND HIP PUSH

Do the beginners version first (page 39), then repeat the exercise twice in 2 counts, and four times in 1 count.

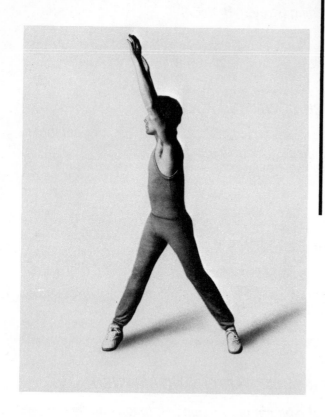

CIRCLE REACH

Description: Keep your legs apart with your feet pointed forward. Start by placing both arms over your head in line with your shoulders. Turn your torso to your right and, in a sweeping circular motion, reach outward away from your hips. Move your body down in a relaxed manner. Continue around toward the left leg, and move through the positions shown in the photos on the opposite side, as you come up from the left to the starting position with your arms upright. Continue around in the same direction four times, and then reverse four times.

Repetitions: Take 4 counts to complete one circle. Do four repetitions to the right and four to the left.

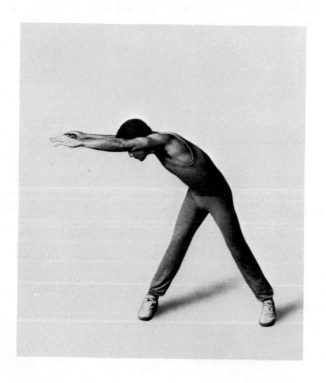

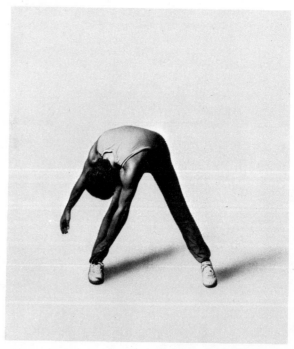

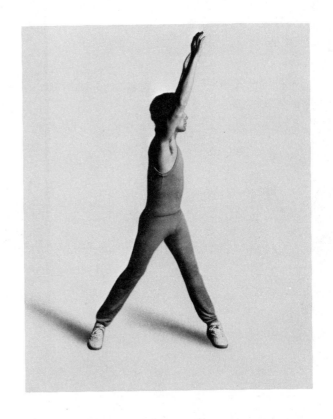

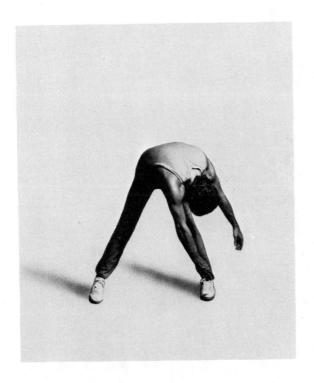

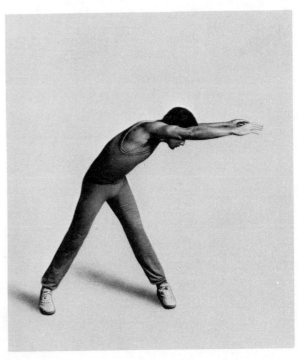

LEG LUNGES

Description & Repetitions: First do the same as the beginners version (page 40). Then bend your right knee, using 4 counts to assume the lunge, and remain down for four easy bounces. Take 4 counts to come up. Repeat with the left leg. Do each side twice in 4 counts and then twice in 2 counts.

PLIÉS IN SECOND AND HEEL LIFTS

Same as the beginners version (page 42).

TURNED-IN JAZZ SECOND

Description: Continuing from the plié in second, lift left heel off the floor and pivot the ball of the left foot until the knee is in a turned-in position. Hold arms straight out to side with palms of the hands facing front and fingers open. Holding this position, extend left hip to left side as far as you can and then to the right side.

Repeat exercise to right side with the right leg.

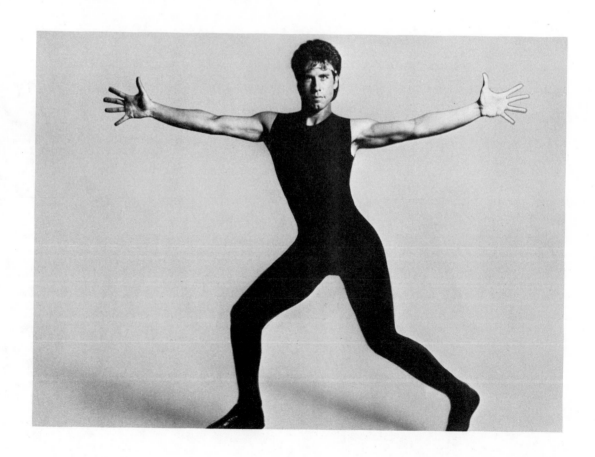

Repetitions: Take 4 counts to bend both legs in second-position plié, 4 counts to lift left heel up, 4 counts to turn left knee in, 2 counts to extend hip to the left and 2 counts to extend hip to the right. Do a total of eight times. Then repeat exercises on right leg.

Note: Remember to keep the heel off the floor while doing the hip extensions. Take 4 counts to turn knee back to starting position, then set heel down and stand normally.

STRETCH AND SQUAT

First do the same as the beginners version (page 44), then repeat the exercise twice in 2 counts and twice in 1 count.

OPEN SIDE SPLIT

Same as the beginners (page 46).

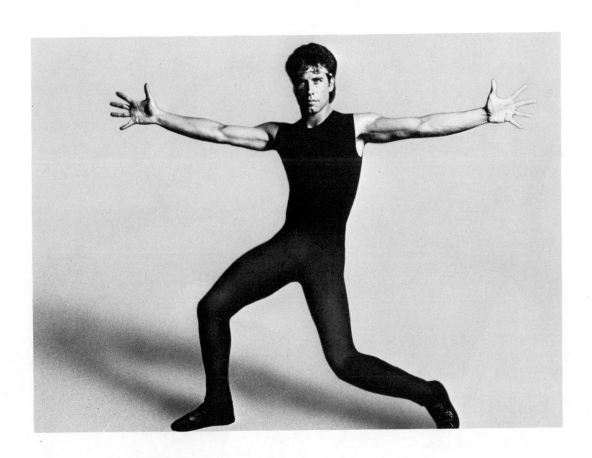

Standing Stretch

ADVANCED
APPROXIMATELY EIGHT MINUTES

REACHING STRETCH

Same as the beginners (page 35).

SIDE STRETCH

Same as the intermediate (page 47).

FORWARD STRETCH AND HIP PUSH

Same as the intermediate (page 47).

Now add this exercise:

TWO-ARM SIDE STRETCH

Description: This exercise is similar to the Side Stretch, but now you reach both arms out to the right side as you bend. Then, from the side position, slowly twist your body so your chest is facing the floor, with both arms still reaching outward. Now drop your arms down and relax your body into a rounded position, placing your nose down close to

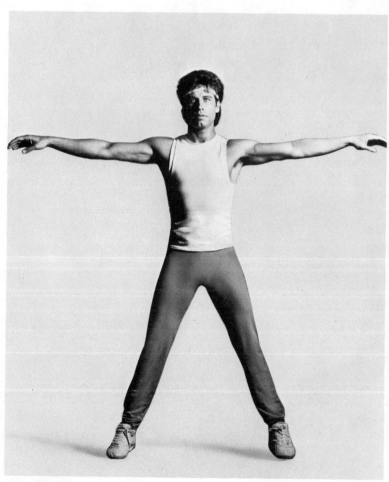

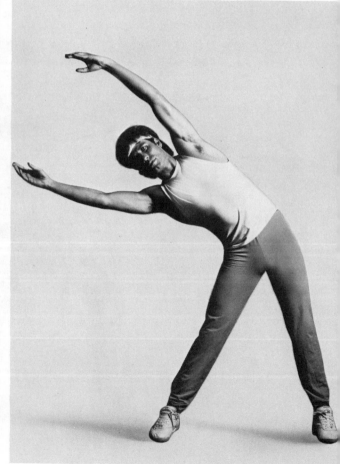

your right knee. From there, reverse the movement, coming back up on the same side. Reach out to the right with your chest facing the floor, then slowly twist to the right side, stretch, and then slowly come back to the upright position. Your arms should start and finish straight out to the side.

Repetitions: Use 4 counts for each movement: 4 counts to bend to the side, 4 counts to twist, 4 counts to place your nose on your knee, 4 counts to reach out, 4 counts to twist to face front, and 4 counts to return to the starting position. Repeat to the left. Then repeat each side, using 2 counts for each movement.

CIRCLE REACH

Same as the intermediate (page 48).

LEG LUNGES

Same as the beginners (page 40).

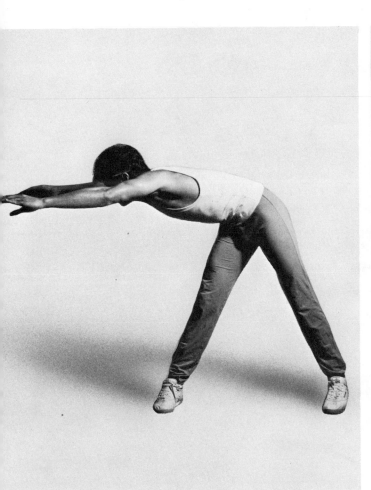

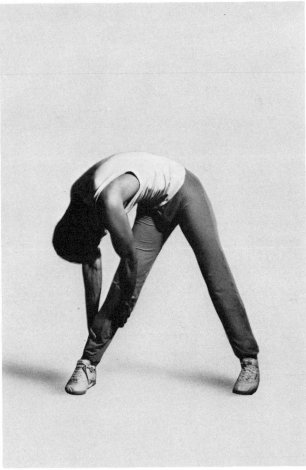

Now add this exercise:

FULL LUNGE SQUAT

Description: This lunge is a continuation of the regular Leg Lunge (page 40). Here you bend your right knee into the lunge and then continue down, sliding your left leg to the side, until you can place your hands on the floor in front of you. Your tail bone will be resting near your right foot. Then, without coming up, move through the center position and transfer your weight to the left leg, to complete the exercise by coming up on the left side through the same positions in reverse.

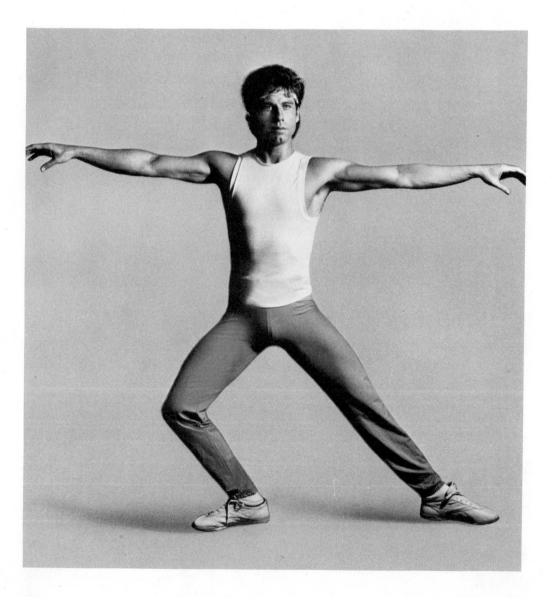

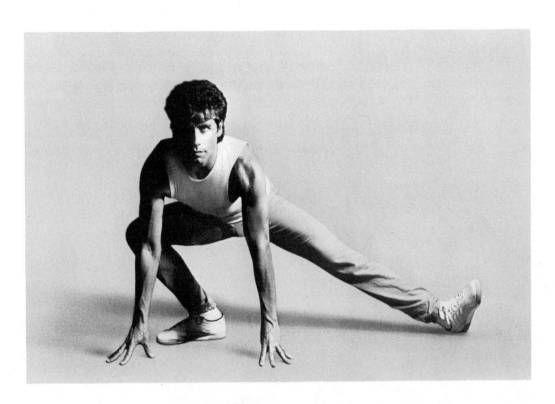

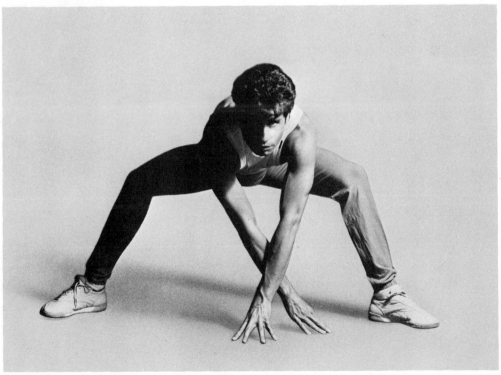

(Exercise continued on next page)

55

Repetitions: Take 8 counts to get from your starting position to the Full Lunge Squat. Then use 8 counts to transfer your body weight to the left leg. Move back to the right leg in 8 counts, then back to the left leg in 8 counts. Then come up the left side to the starting position.

Note: When you have finished the Full Lunge Squat, take a moment to shake your legs out.

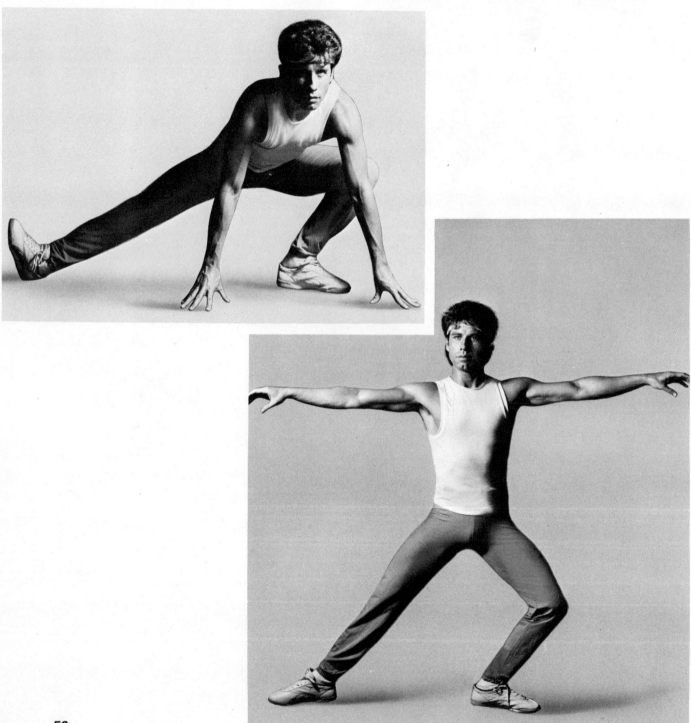

PLIÉS IN SECOND AND HEEL LIFTS

Same as the beginners version (page 42).

TURNED-IN JAZZ SECOND

Same as the intermediate version (page 50).

STRETCH AND SQUAT

Same as the intermediate version (page 51).

OPEN SIDE SPLIT

Same as the beginners version (page 46).

Floor Stretch

BEGINNERS
APPROXIMATELY SIX MINUTES

Starting Position: Sit on the floor with your legs together straight out in front of you. Rest your hands on the floor to your sides and keep your back in a straight upright position with your shoulders relaxed and your stomach muscles lifted.

Note: *The muscles supporting your spine need to be exercised. Your back will not stay in a straight upright position without continuous effort.*

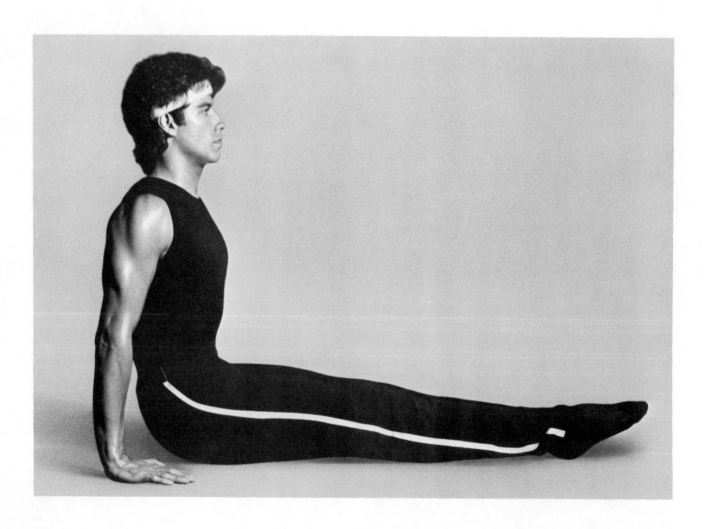

FLEX AND POINT

This exercise works the Achilles tendon and gives the ankles mobility.

Description: Start by pointing your toes while keeping your legs and ankles together. Curl your toes up toward your chest, then press your insteps and toes down to point your feet.

Repetitions: Do four flex-and-points, using 2 counts to flex and 2 counts to point. Then do four more repetitions, using only 1 count to flex and 1 count to point.

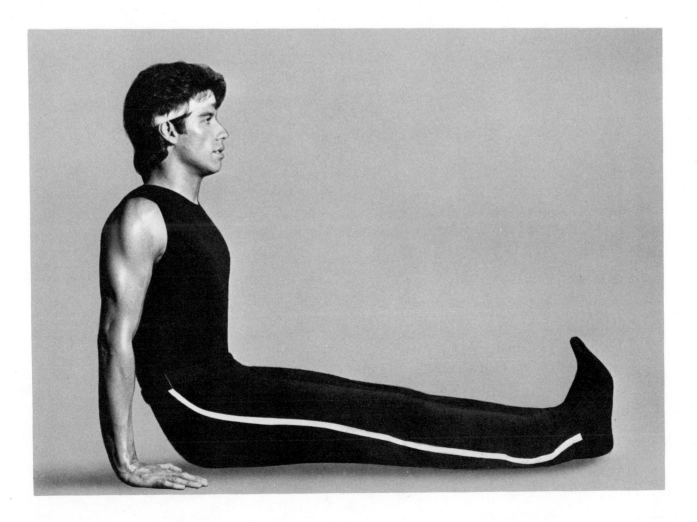

FORWARD STRETCH

This exercise stretches the hamstring and back muscles.

Description: After the Flex and Point exercise, hold your feet in a flexed position. Reach both arms forward so they are parallel to your legs, and bounce gently on each count, keeping your back straight. Then point the feet, round your back by dropping your head down, grab your ankles with your hands, and gently pull.

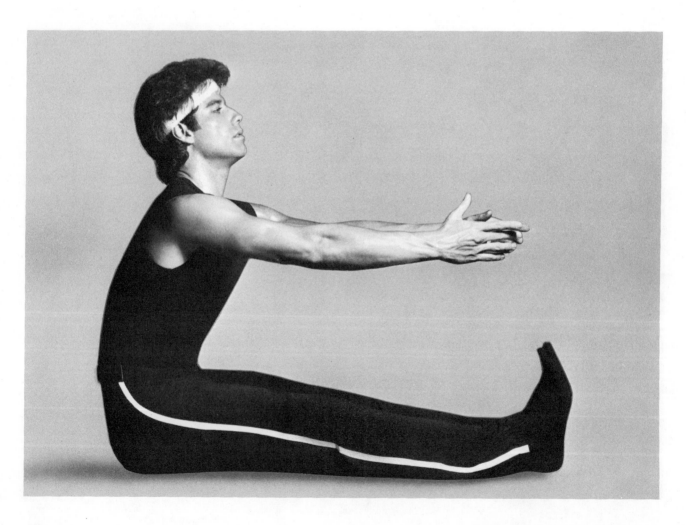

Repetitions: Use 8 counts to reach forward bouncing gently with the feet flexed, and 8 counts to round and pull your head down. Repeat using 4 counts, then 2 counts, and then use 1 count four times.

On the fourth 1-count, hold your head down close to your knees for one long continuous stretch as you count to eight.

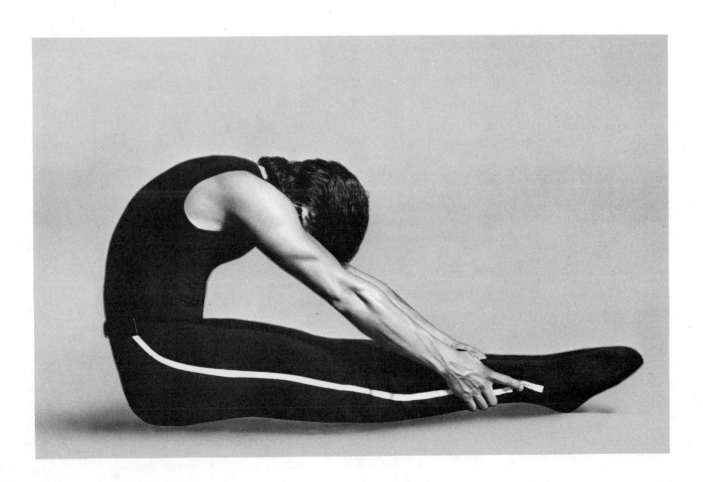

JAZZ LOTUS AND CONTRACT AND ARCH

This works the hip joint area and stretches the back muscles and spine.

Description: In a sitting position, bring the soles of your feet together with your legs turned out so your knees are close to the floor. Hold on to your ankles with your hands. Lift your back up as straight as you can get it. You will need to use your ankles as a brace to pull against to get your spine straight. Begin by releasing your back into a rounded, contracted state and drop your chin to your chest. Then bend over from your waist and place your head as close to your feet as possible. Using your ankles as a brace, pull your head forward, stretching your spine as straight as possible, and slowly lift yourself into an upright sitting position.

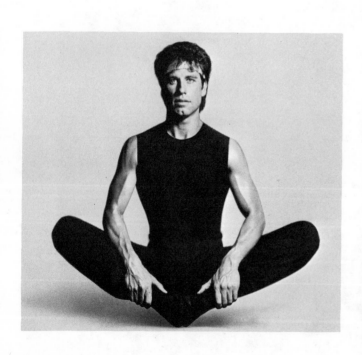

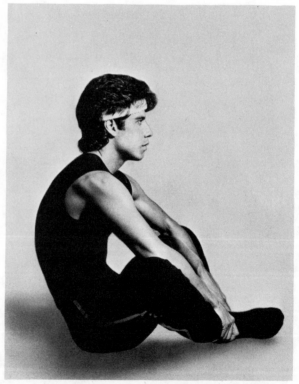

Repetitions: Take 8 counts to contract downward, and 8 counts to reach out and come up to a straight position. Do this twice in 8 counts and then twice in 4 counts.

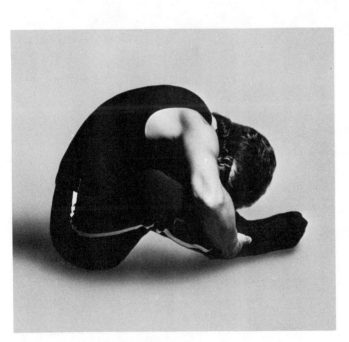

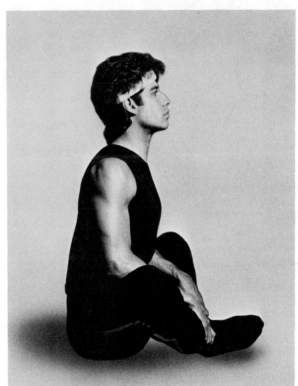

Changing Position: After completing the previous exercise, keep your legs in the same position and lie back on the floor. Relax totally, your knees open to the side, and let gravity work. Stay relaxed in this position for 16 counts, and then extend your legs straight on the floor so you are now completely flat on your back.

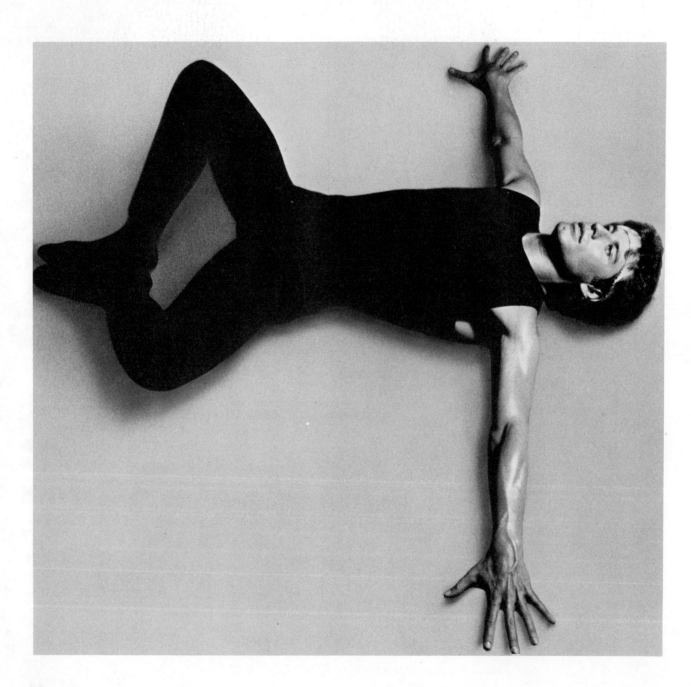

KNEE AND LEG PULLS

This stretches your hamstrings and split position.

Description: Bend your right knee up to your chest and clasp it with both hands. Apply a gentle pulling pressure while keeping your right hip down on the floor. Then grab behind the leg with your hands and slowly straighten it, keeping your leg as close to your chest as possible. With the leg straight do a series of pulls, bringing it even closer to your chest. Slowly release the right leg down to the floor. Then do the same with the left leg.

Repetitions: Take 4 counts to complete each of the three parts: Pull your knee up to your chest, grab it and slowly extend leg straight in 4 counts. (During this part of the exercise, make sure you use all 4 counts to get your leg straight. Your leg shouldn't be completely straight until the fourth count.) With the leg straight pull for 4 counts, and then let it down to the floor in 4 counts. It should touch the floor on the fourth count. Do each leg once taking 4 counts for each movement, once taking 2 counts for each movement, and twice taking 1 count.

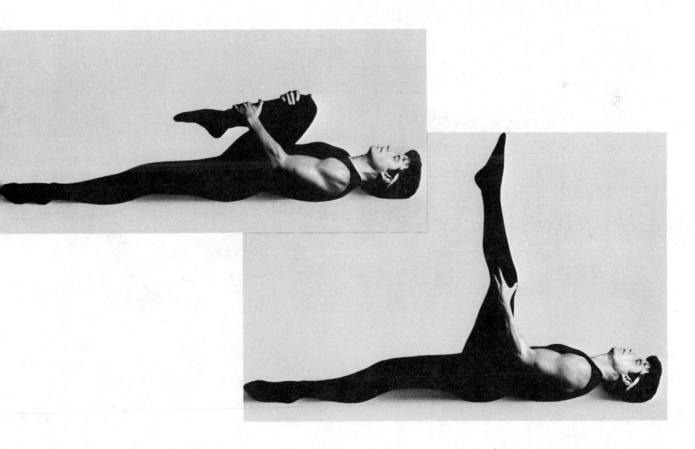

EXTEND AND OPEN SIDE

This stretches the inside leg muscles and hamstrings.

Description: Remain on your back. Bring both your knees up to your chest in a bent position. Keep your tail bone on the floor and feel your knees and ankles pressing together as you keep your feet pointed. Begin by extending your legs straight up to a vertical position, then open your legs out to the side as far as you can, still keeping your legs straight. Apply a little extra pressure with your hands to get your legs even farther apart. Then bring them back together, keeping them straight, and bend them back to the starting position.

Repetitions: Take 4 counts to complete each movement: 4 counts to extend, 4 counts to open, 4 counts back together, and 4 counts to bend knees to chest. Do this twice in 4 counts and then twice in 2 counts.

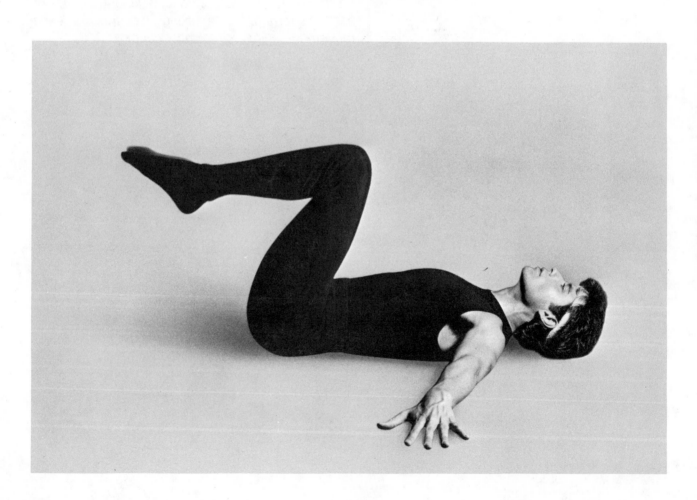

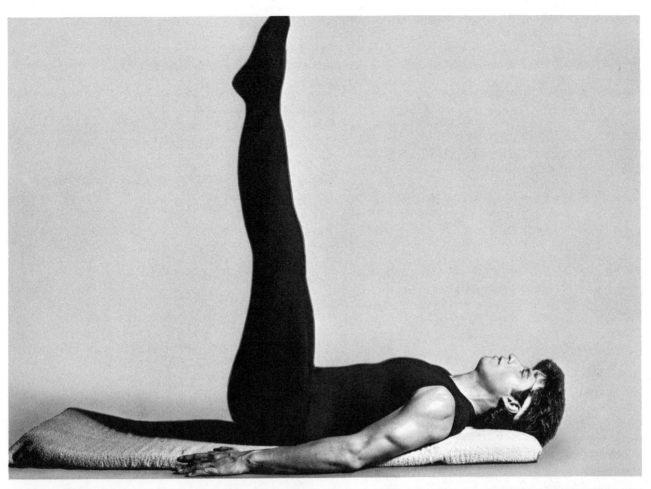

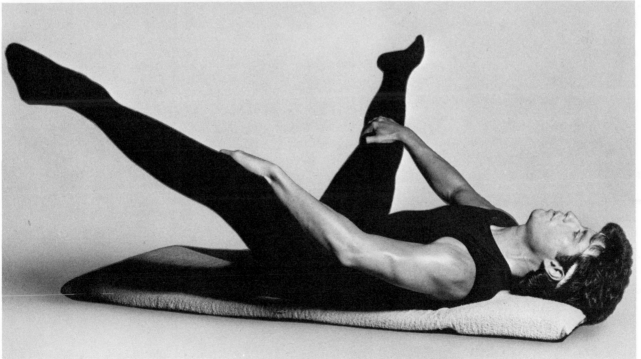

LEG LOWER

This exercise strengthens your stomach muscles and works the back as well.

Description: *Sit up on your tail bone with your elbows resting on the floor for support. Bring your knees up to your chest. Try to keep your back straight and your shoulders down. Begin by extending your legs up in a vertical position. Then slowly lower your legs toward the floor. Keep your legs straight and your feet pointed. If this is extremely difficult, you may bend your knees slightly until you gain the stretch and strength to keep them straight. Stop with your feet about two inches off the floor. Then bend your knees up to your chest and begin again.*

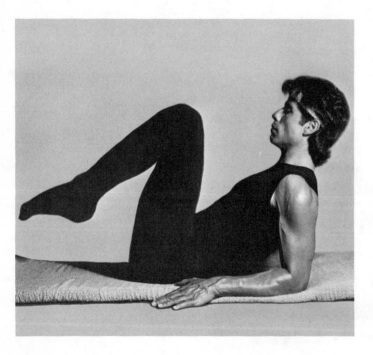

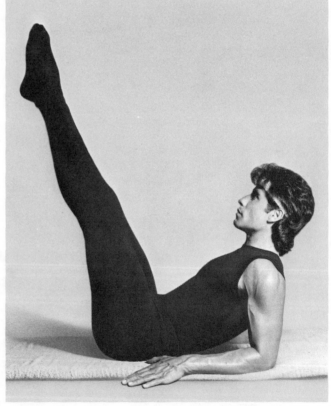

Repetitions: Take 8 counts to lower your legs to the floor. Then when you bend your knees in again, rest for 8 counts. Then repeat. Then use 4 counts with a 4-count rest, twice.

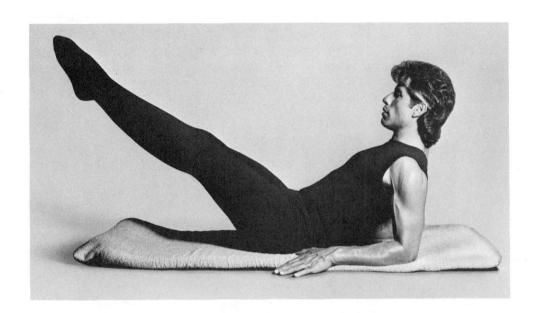

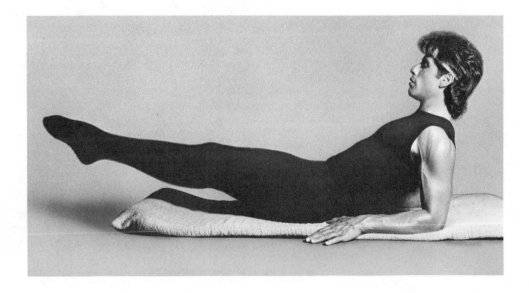

Changing Position: Sit upright and open your legs out to the side as far as you can.

OPEN SPLIT

This stretches the inside leg muscles, increases flexibility in your hips, and stretches your sides and hamstrings.

Description: Sit on the floor and open your legs as wide as you can. Flex your feet, sit up straight, and reach your arms straight out in front of you at about shoulder width. Begin by doing easy bounces forward, keeping your back straight and feet flexed. Then reach over to the right leg and pull your head down to your right knee. Repeat, reaching over to the left leg.

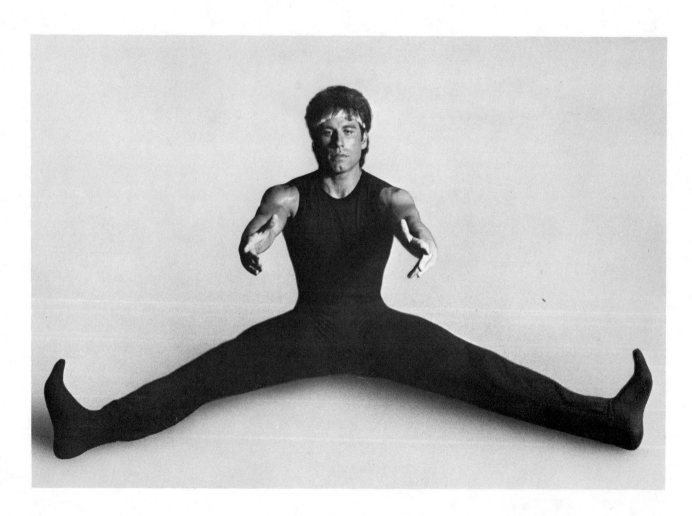

Repetitions: Do eight bounces forward, then eight bounces to the right leg, and then eight bounces to the left leg. Then do four bounces for each move. Then do two bounces.

After completing this exercise, sit up straight again, flex both feet and reach both arms forward. Reach as far forward as possible with your back as straight as can be. Do this in 8 counts. Then relax forward, dropping your head and rounding your back for 8 counts. Work to get your chest on the floor. Take it in stages. First put your hands on the floor, then your elbows, then your nose, and then your chest.

Do this twice.

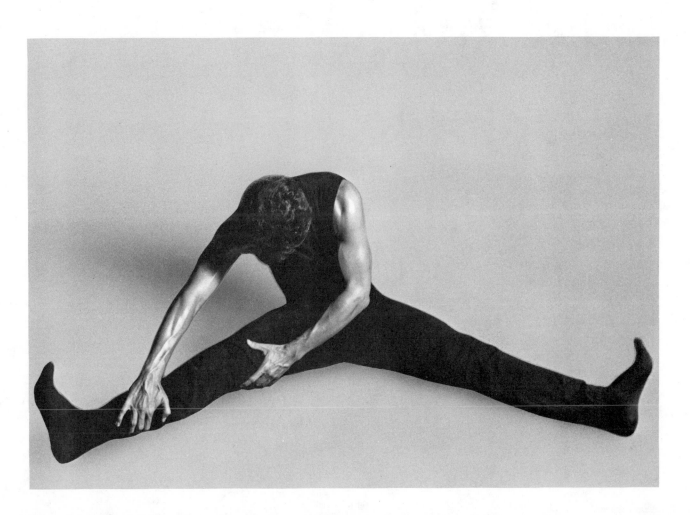

YOGA TWIST

This exercise stretches your spine and back muscles as well as your upper thigh and buttocks.

Description: *Assume a sitting position with both legs bent. Bring your left foot close to your body, with your outer thigh and calf resting on the floor. Cross your right leg over your left, your right foot flat*

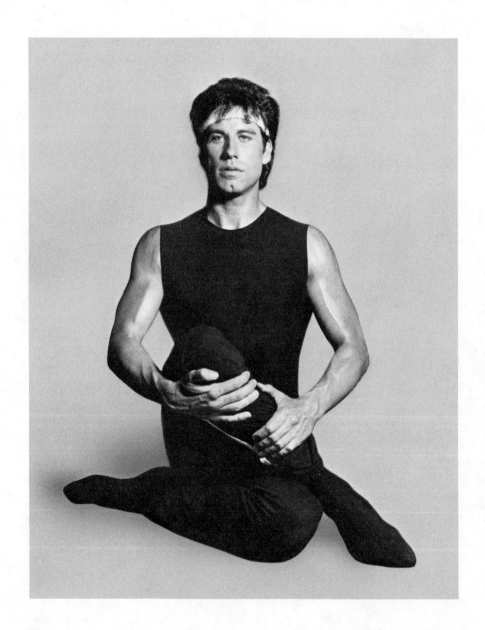

on the floor. Your right knee will be pointing up to the ceiling. Then hold on to your right leg with your left arm and lift your back straight, bracing yourself with your right hand on the floor. Twist your back and spine to the right, applying a gentle pressure against your right knee with your left arm.

Repetitions: Stretch in this position for 8 counts.

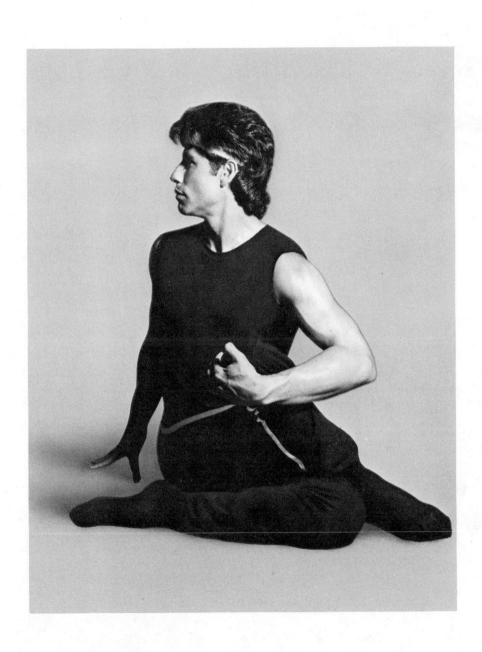

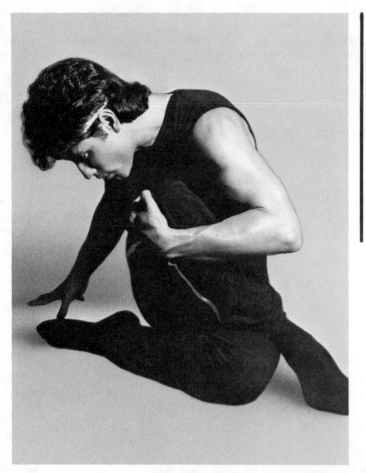

Description: Without changing position drop your head down and round your back in a relaxed manner. Slowly move your body to the front, still keeping your head down. Then lift your back up as straight as you can and hold on to your right knee with both hands to brace and help pull your back straight. When you lift your back up, keep your shoulders relaxed and down. Then change legs so the left leg is crossed over the right, and repeat.

Repetitions: Hold the twist with head dropped for 8 counts. Hold the front position with head dropped for 8 counts. Pull your back straight for 8 counts. Repeat on other side.

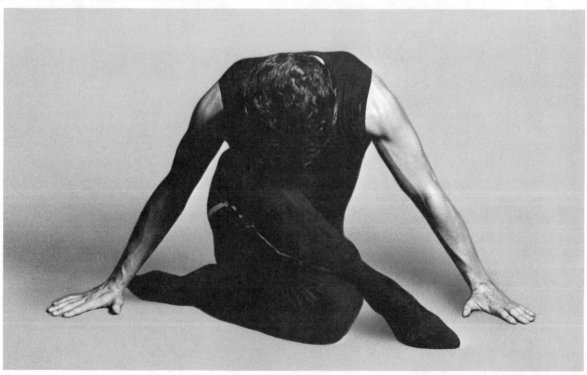

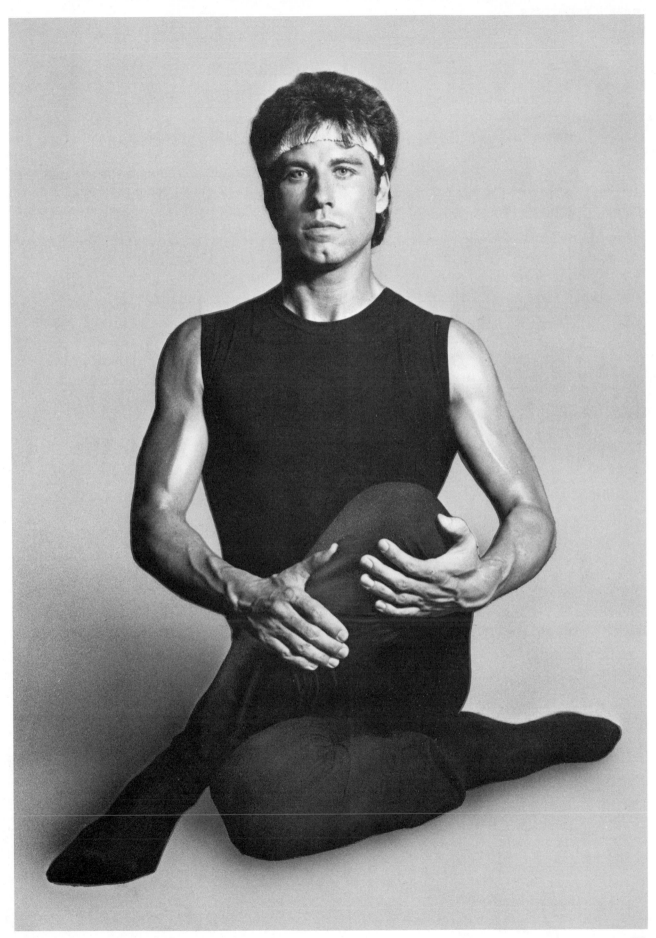

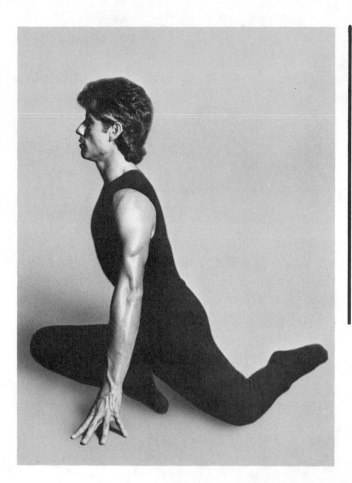

BENT CROSS STRETCH

This exercise is great for preparing to do a split.

Description: *Sit on the floor with your right leg in front and both legs bent as in the photograph. Your hands are resting on the floor at your sides. Start with your back upright. Hold the straight-back position, then drop your head down to the floor, relaxing and rounding your back. Leaving your head down, straighten your back leg directly behind you. Then, keeping your back leg straight and bracing your hands on the floor, lift your back up straight and drop your head back as far as you can.*

Repetitions: *Take 8 counts for the straight-back position, 8 counts for the round-back position, 8 counts to straighten your back leg, and 8 counts to lift and stretch your head back.*

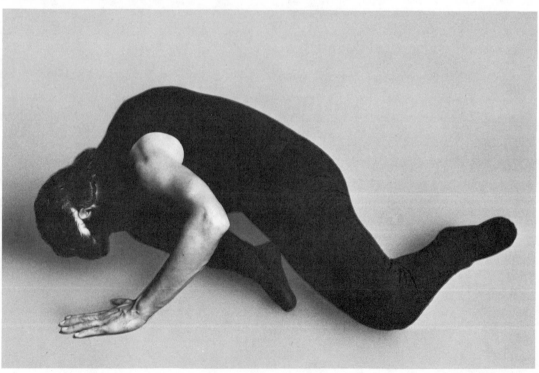

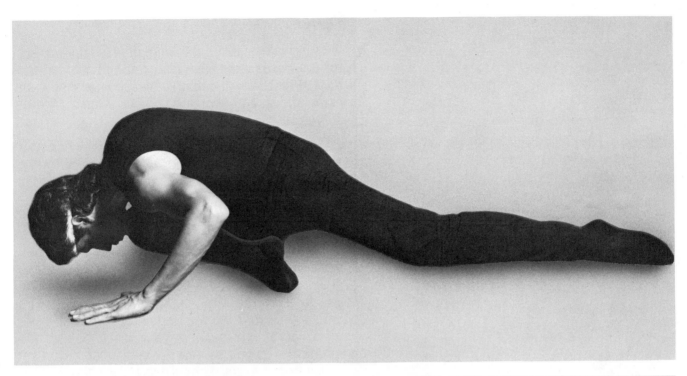

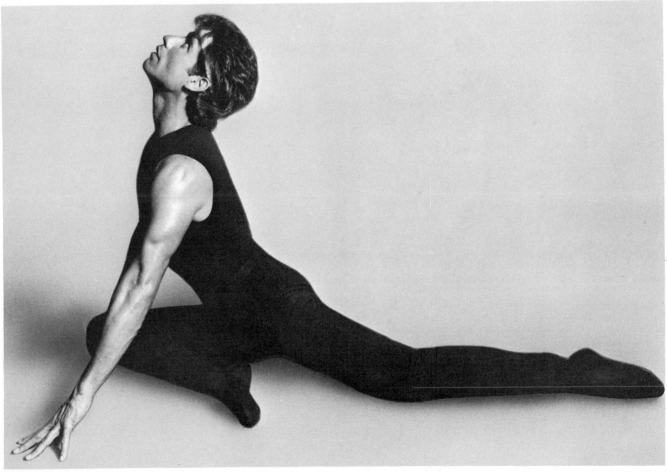

LUNGE AND SPLIT

Working into a split is the ultimate accomplishment for the dance exerciser. Take care not to push too hard at first. A split can only be accomplished after many months of working. Below, Marilu Henner shows how it is done.

Description: *Kneel on your left knee, with your right leg forward, bent, foot flat on the floor. Keep your right leg turned out so your right knee is pointing to the right side. Take 8 counts to lean your weight forward and turn your right knee out. Keep your stomach muscles lifted. Keep your right knee in line with your right foot as you are bending. Then place your hands on the floor in front of you and straighten your left leg behind you, the ball of the left foot on the floor and your left knee facing downward. Your left leg should be in direct alignment with your spine. Keep your right knee bent and turned out as you do eight easy bounces, working your left hip to the floor. Then point your left foot*

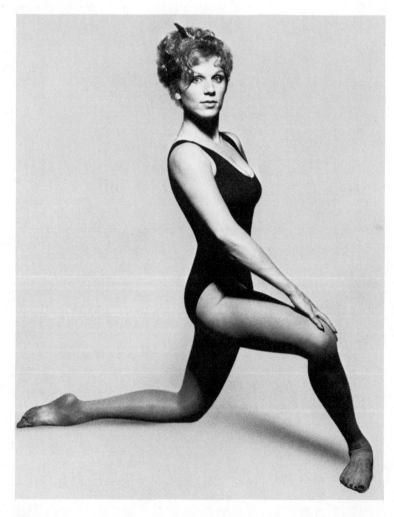

and slide it back, straightening your right leg as you go into as much of a split as possible. Remember not to push yourself too far at first. When you slide back into the split you can bend your back knee to ease some of the pressure.

Repetitions: After completing the exercise once, reverse sides and repeat with the right leg.

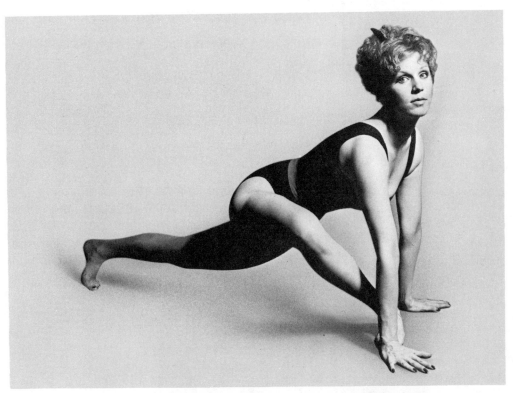

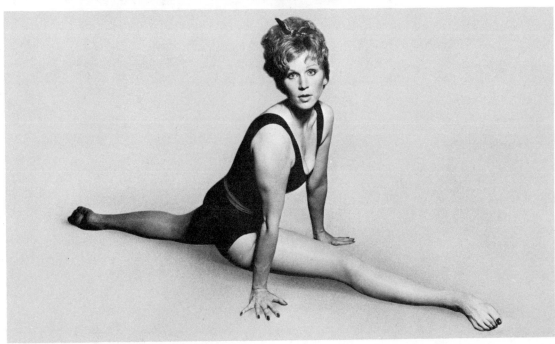

Floor Stretch

INTERMEDIATE
APPROXIMATELY EIGHT MINUTES

FLEX AND POINT

Same as the beginners (page 59).

FORWARD STRETCH

Same as the beginners (page 60).

JAZZ LOTUS AND CONTRACT AND ARCH

Same as the beginners (page 62).

Now add this new exercise:

INNER THIGH SQUEEZE

This exercise works the inner thigh muscles and the back and spine.

Starting Position: Immediately after completing the Jazz Lotus exercise, bring your legs together so your knees touch. Keep your feet flat on the floor and sit up on your tail bone. Hold your legs together with both arms wrapped around them. Lift your back as straight as you can.

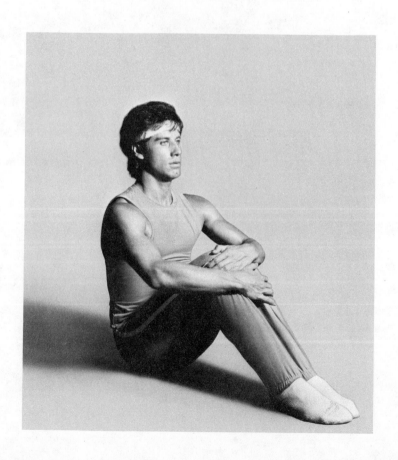

Description: Extend right arm straight out to the side. Then extend left arm. Both arms are now extended. When you release your arms your knees will want to separate. Work to keep them pressed together. Grasp your legs again for a second, then let your knees fall open to the Jazz Lotus position (soles of the feet together) and relax your head down with your back rounded. Then lift your back up and bring your knees together again.

Repetitions: Hold the starting position for 8 counts. Extend your arms and hold for 8 counts. Hold in the relaxed position with your head down for 8 counts. Take 8 counts to lift your back up to the starting position. Then repeat exercise.

Now continue to the Changing Position described in the beginners stretch on page 64.

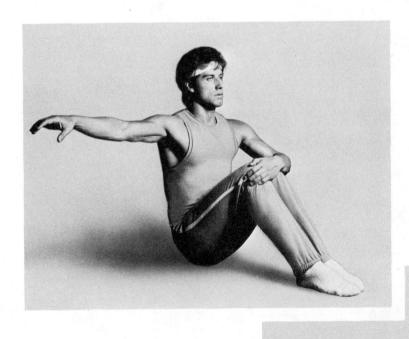

KNEE AND LEG PULLS

Same as the beginners (page 65).

OPEN SPLIT ON BACK AND HOLD

This is a variation of the Extend and Open Side stretch described in the beginners floor stretch (page 66).

Description: Resting on your back, extend your legs straight up toward the ceiling. Open them out to the side and flex your feet so that your toes are pointing downward. Apply extra pressure with your hands. Keeping the backs of your legs straight, slowly bring your legs together and point your feet, then slowly open your legs to the side again and flex your feet.

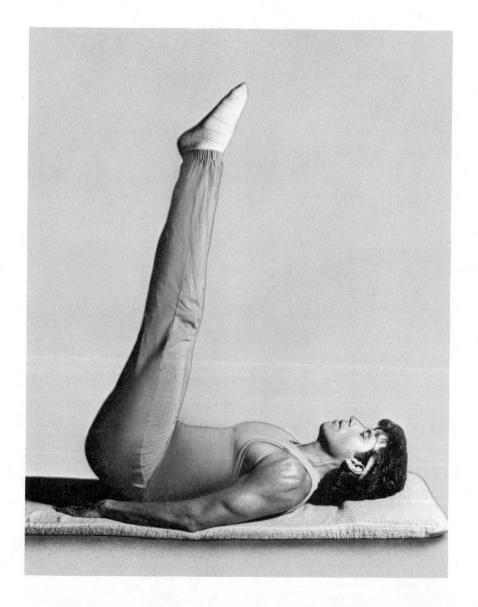

Repetitions: Begin by holding the open position for a total of 16 counts. Use your hands on the insides of your knees and apply a gentle pressure. Then use 4 counts to bring your legs together, pointing your feet, and 4 counts to open to the side, flexing. Do this twice using 4 counts, then twice using 2 counts to bring your legs together and 2 counts to open.

Changing Position: After completing the Open Split, change positions by bringing your legs together. Bend them to your chest and lift your shoulders and head, balancing on your elbows, so your weight is resting on your tail bone (see page 68).

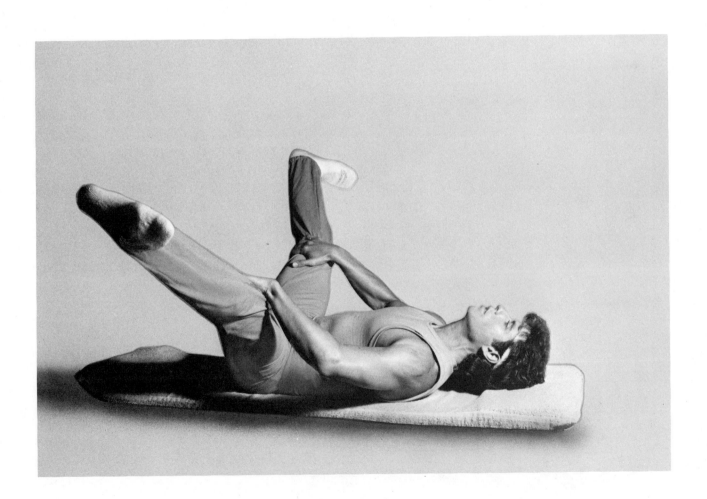

LEG LOWER

Do the exercise as described in the beginners stretch (page 68), and then add to it the following.

Description & Repetitions: *Start with your legs extended vertically upward. Take 4 counts to lower your legs to an inch off the floor. This time, without bending your legs, bring them back up in 4 counts to the starting vertical position. Do this a total of four times.*

   Note: *It will be hard to bring your legs back up without bending them. It is this kind of effort that brings results in tightening and toning the stomach muscles.*

   After completing this exercise, lie on your back with your legs straight on the floor and relax for 16 counts.
   Now do this new exercise:

HIP THRUST

This exercise is perfect for tightening the buttocks and stomach muscles.

Description: *While still lying down, bend your knees and put your feet flat on the floor twelve inches apart, with your knees pointing straight up.*

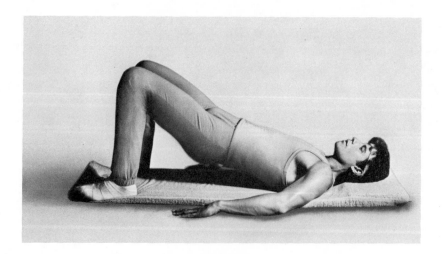

Keep your arms down by your sides. Begin by lifting your hips off the floor. Your feet should remain flat— you will now be resting on your upper back, shoulders, and neck. Push your hips up to the ceiling in a bouncing fashion, releasing your hips down an inch or two between each thrust. Then hold the thrust position with your buttocks held tight.

Repetitions: Do the hip thrust 8 times, using 1 count for each push, and then hold in the thrust position for 4 counts. Repeat this entire sequence a total of four times.

After this, sit up and continue.

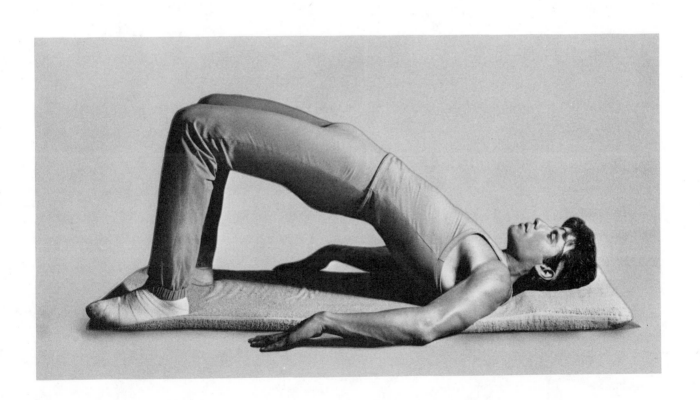

OPEN SPLIT

Description: Sit on the floor and open your legs as wide as you can, as Marilu is doing below. Point your toes, sit up straight, and open your arms directly out to the side. Begin by extending your left arm over your head as you lean and stretch to the right side. Your right arm will stretch out to the right. Then twist your body, holding your right ankle, and bend forward until your head touches your knee. Twist back to the side position and slowly come up to the center position with your back straight and your arms to the sides. Then repeat the exercise going to the left.

Repetitions: Use 8 counts on each stretch: 8 counts side, 8 counts to face the leg, 8 counts back to the side, and 8 counts to come up. Repeat to the left using 8 counts. Then repeat both sides using only 4 counts for each stretch.

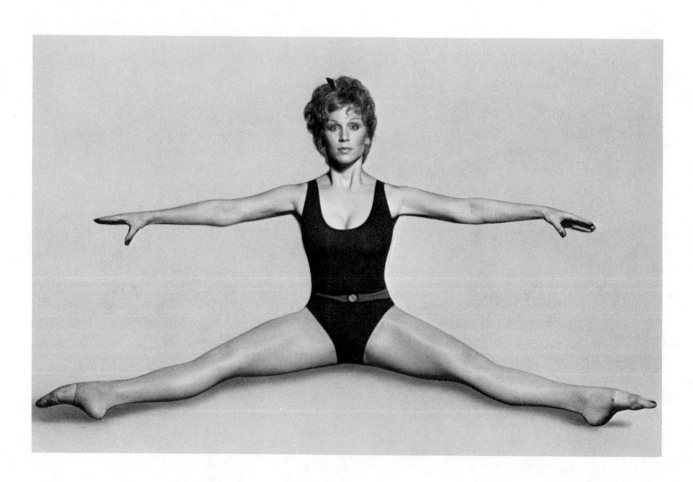

YOGA TWIST

Same as beginners (page 72).

BENT CROSS STRETCH

Same as beginners (page 76).

LUNGE AND SPLIT

Same as beginners (page 78).

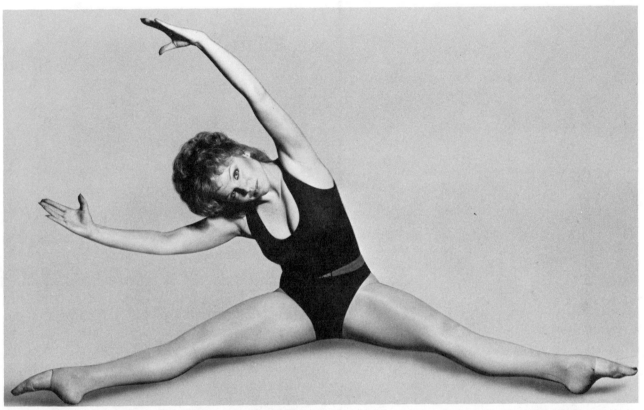

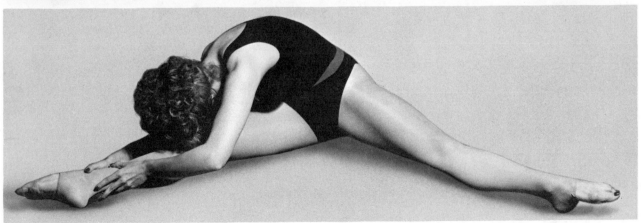

Floor Stretch

ADVANCED
APPROXIMATELY NINE MINUTES

FLEX AND POINT

Same as the beginners (page 59).

FORWARD STRETCH

Same as the beginners (page 60).

JAZZ LOTUS AND CONTRACT AND ARCH

Same as the beginners (page 62).

INNER THIGH SQUEEZE

Same as the intermediate (page 80).

KNEE AND LEG PULLS

Same as the beginners (page 65).

Now do this new exercise:

BACK AND HAMSTRING STRETCH

This one is great for stretching your spine and back muscles. It also stretches the Achilles tendon and hamstrings, and brings the blood up to your head.

Description: Lying on your back after completing the Knee and Leg Pulls as above, bend both your legs to your chest with your knees together and feet pointed. Then straighten your legs over your head behind you. Flex your feet and try to place the balls of your feet on the floor. You may not be able to get your feet to touch the floor. That's okay, just get them as close to the floor as you can. Then bend your knees and place them by your ears, as close to the floor as possible. Throughout the exercise keep your arms down by your sides.

Repetitions: Place your feet over your head and flexed on the floor for 8 counts. Then bend your knees to your ears for 8 counts. Then repeat. Next, take 4 counts for each movement, twice.

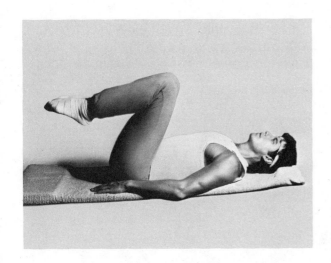

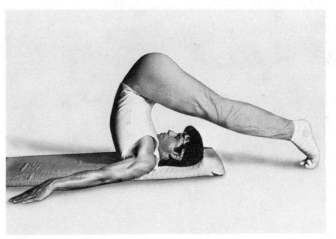

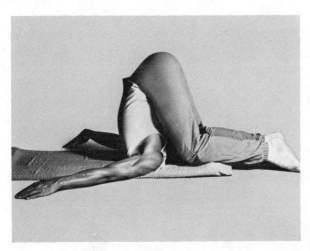

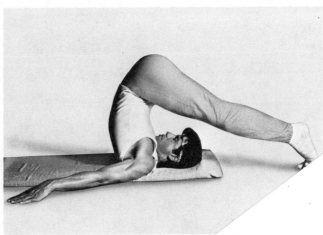

Now take 16 counts to roll slowly down your spine until your tail bone is on the floor. Try to feel one vertebra at a time releasing down to the floor.

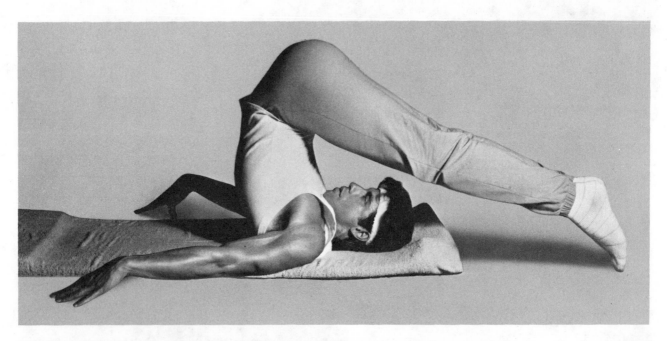

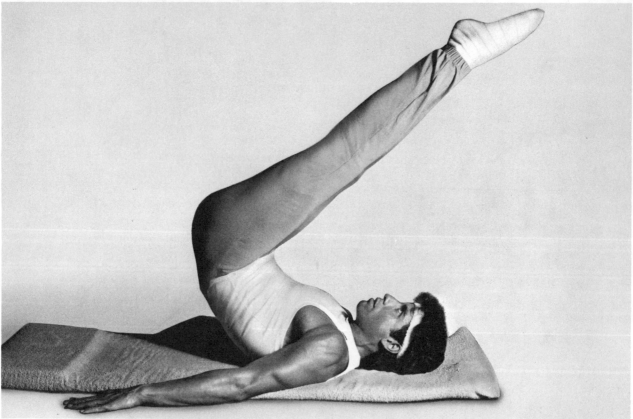

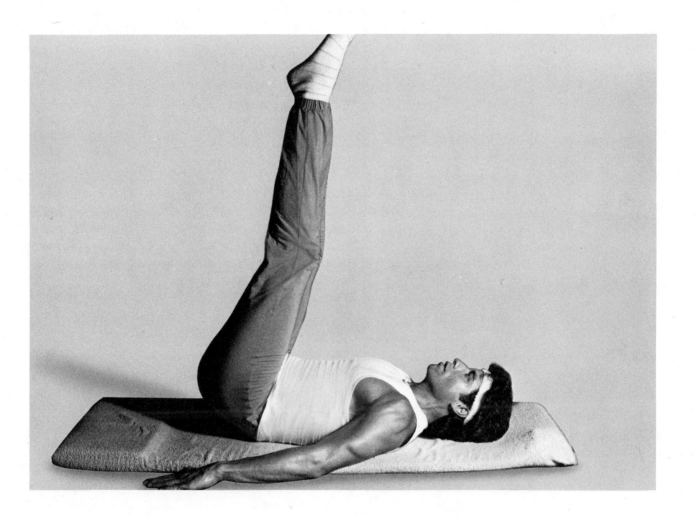

OPEN SPLIT ON BACK AND HOLD

Same as the intermediate stretch (page 82).

LEG LOWER

Same as the intermediate stretch (page 84).

HIP THRUST

Same as the intermediate stretch (page 85).

Now add this new exercise:

BACKBEND ARCH

A great counter stretch to the preceding stomach-tightening exercises. It also stretches the spine and back.

Description: *Remain lying on your back, and keep your knees bent, feet flat on the floor and about twelve inches apart. Place your hands, palms down, on the floor by your ears, fingers pointing toward your shoulders. Then push yourself up off the floor as high as you can. Let your head relax backward and look down to the floor, letting your heels push off the floor. Do not overdo this at first. You need not straighten your arms until you are ready.*

Repetitions: *Do only one of these, holding at the top of the arch for 8 counts. Then release yourself down slowly, watching out so you don't hit your head.*

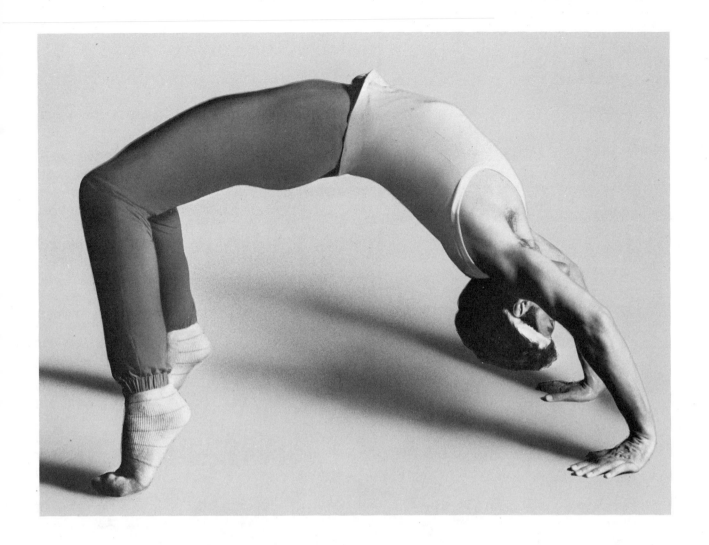

Now sit up and continue.

OPEN SPLIT
Same as the intermediate stretch (page 86).

YOGA TWIST
Same as the beginners stretch (page 72).

Now add this new exercise:

PUSH UP–BACK ARCH

This stretches the spine and tightens the upper back, thigh, and buttocks.

Description: Turn over onto your stomach with your legs on the floor. Place your hands on the floor next to your shoulders. Now push your back up off the floor by straightening your arms. Push up as high as you can without lifting your hip bones off the floor or letting your shoulders hunch up. Unless you are very loose in the spine you should not straighten your arms all the way. As you push up, stop if you feel your shoulders starting to hunch. Concentrate on keeping your shoulders down by pulling your shoulder blades down.

Repetitions: Use 4 counts to push yourself up, stay up for 4 counts, then take 4 counts to come down slowly. Repeat once more.

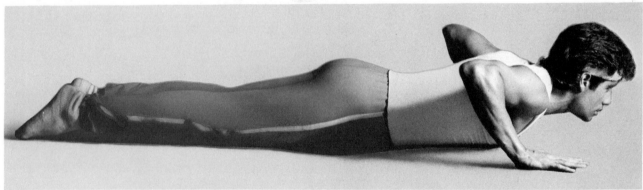

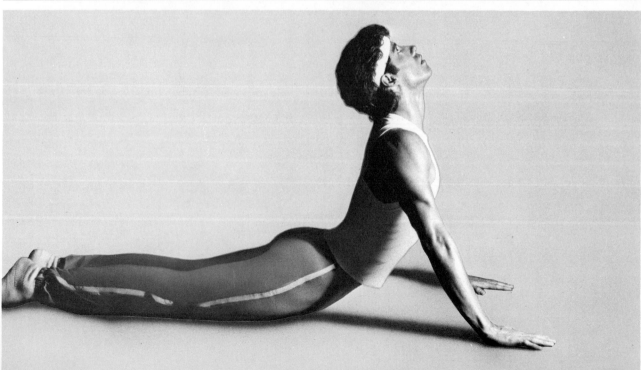

Description: Then stretch your arms out to your sides and separate your legs about one foot. Arch your back up, lifting your back and legs off the ground as high as you can, as in a swan dive. You will be balancing on your hip bones.

Repetitions: Take 4 counts to go up and 4 counts to come down. Be sure not to jerk yourself up to the swan arch. Use the counts to go up slowly and release yourself down slowly. Do this part of the exercise twice.

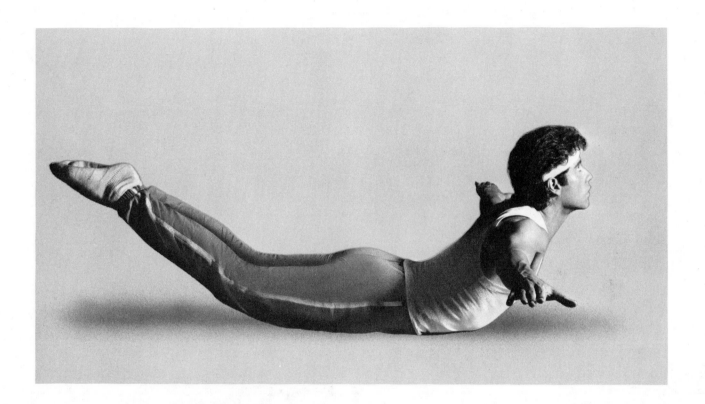

Now change your position back to do:

BENT CROSS STRETCH

Same as beginners (page 76).

LUNGE AND SPLIT

Same as the beginners (page 78).

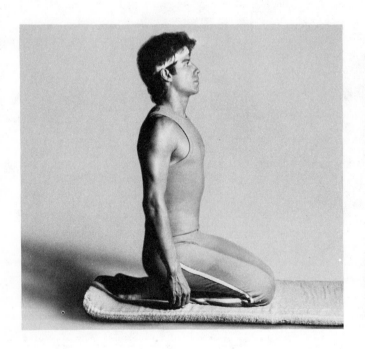

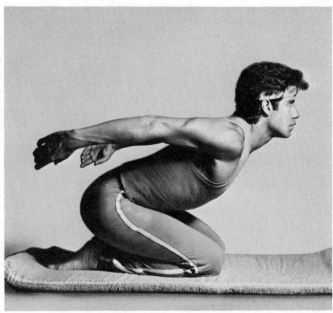

KNEE ARCH AND ROLL-UP

Description: Kneel with your tail bone resting on your heels. You will feel your thighs stretching. Begin by arching your back forward as you bring your chest down to your knees. Hold your head up as you descend. At the bottom of the movement drop your head and round your back. Then slowly roll up, keeping your chin on your chest until you are completely upright.

Repetitions: Take 8 counts to arch forward and 8 counts to roll up. Repeat in 8 counts—then do twice in 4 counts.

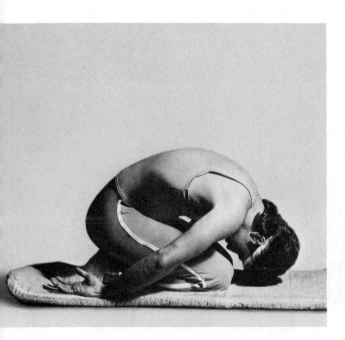
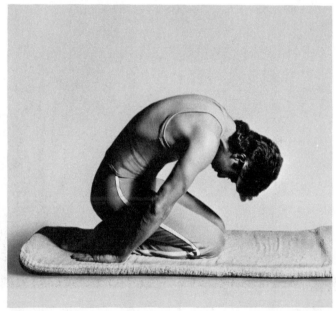

Standing Stretch Finish

*BEGINNERS
APPROXIMATELY FIVE MINUTES*

Now is the time to bring out your chair for assistance.

PLIÉS (knee bends)

These develop overall leg strength. They stretch the Achilles tendon and make you conscious of your back alignment and balance.

Description: Place the chair directly in front of you with the back toward you. Hold on to the top of the back and stand far enough away so your knees don't hit the chair when you bend. Place your feet tight together in a parallel position. You will do two

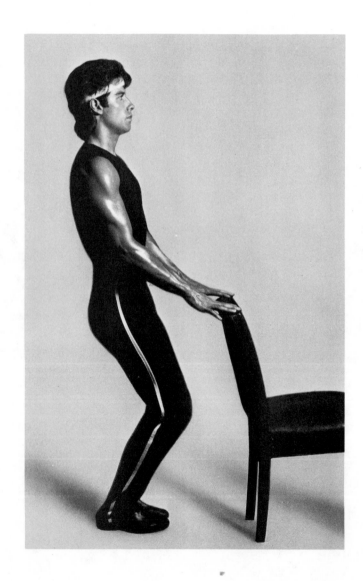

demi-pliés and then two grand pliés. In the demi- or half plié you go halfway down when bending, keeping your heels on the floor. As you bend do not let your hips release back so that your buttocks are sticking out. Keep your stomach lifted. Imagine you are wearing a girdle that's holding your stomach in. In the grand or deep plié you go all the way down so that your heels come off the floor and your tail bone rests on your heels for a moment.

Repetitions: Take 2 counts to do the demi-plié and 2 counts to come up. Do the demi-plié twice, then do two grand pliés. Take 4 counts to go down and 4 counts to come up.

   Note: *Use the chair for balance and for any help you may need when coming up from the plié. Eventually you want to rely less and less on the chair and more on your own leg strength and balance.*

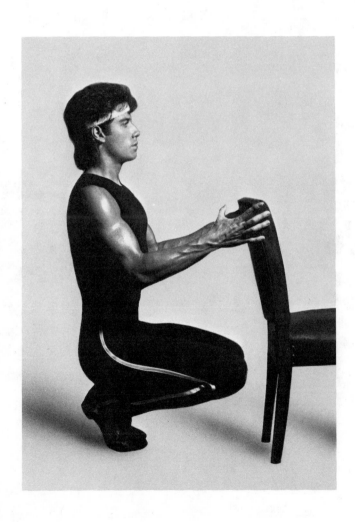

Description: Now turn your feet out in a ballet first position. Your heels should be touching while your feet are pointing outward. Keep your legs together. Do not turn out so far as to strain your knees.

Repetitions: Repeat the same number of demi- and grand pliés with feet turned out as you did with feet parallel. When you do pliés in first position, you should keep your knees pointing in a direct line over your toes.

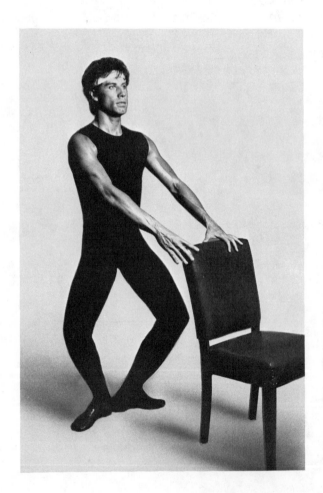
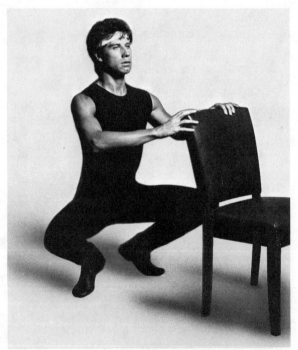

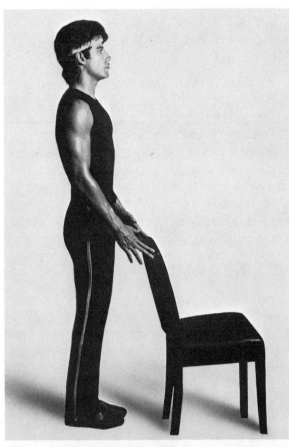

CALF RISES

This strengthens and tightens calves and stretches the Achilles tendon. It also develops your balance.

Description: *Bring your feet back to a parallel position. Keep hold of the back of the chair with your hands. Do one demi-plié, then straighten up, then rise on the balls of your feet, keeping your ankles together. Then lower.*

Repetitions: *Take 2 counts for each movement: 2 counts to do the demi-plié, 2 counts to straighten, 2 counts to rise, and 2 counts to lower. Do this a total of four times. Then repeat four times, using only 1 count for each movement.*

On the fourth repetition of the 1-count, rise and hold the position. You want to get your heels high off the floor and keep your ankles pressed together. Let go of the chair and place your arms directly out to the sides. Balance there, trying not to move your feet, for 8 counts. Take hold of the chair again and slowly ease yourself down.

Now shake your legs out. Remove the chair for the next two exercises.

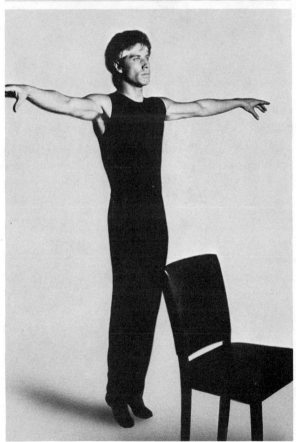

KICKS

These exercises develop mobility of the hip joints and stretch the legs.

Front Kicks Description: Stand on your left leg and place your right foot in a touch position next to the left foot. The touch position is one where the ball of the foot is resting on the floor with little or no weight on it. Now place your arms directly to the sides for balance. Begin by stepping forward on your right leg, then swing your left leg straight up in front of you in a big sweeping kick. (Make sure the kicking leg sweeps up directly in front of your body.) Bring the kicking leg back to the floor behind you, put your weight on it and return the right leg to its starting position.

Repetitions: Each movement should take 1 count. Step forward 1 count, kick 1 count, step back 1 count, and touch together 1 count. Complete four kicks on the left leg. Then change and do four kicks on the right leg.

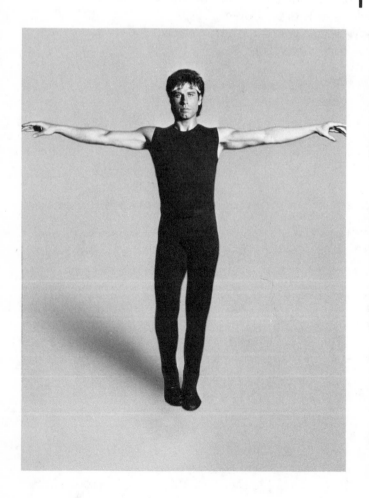
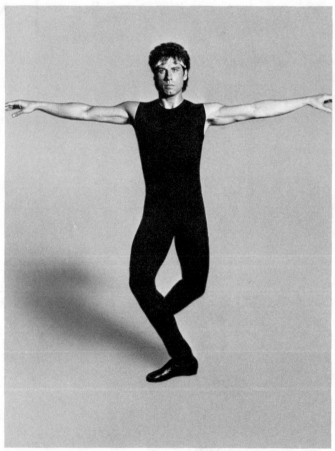

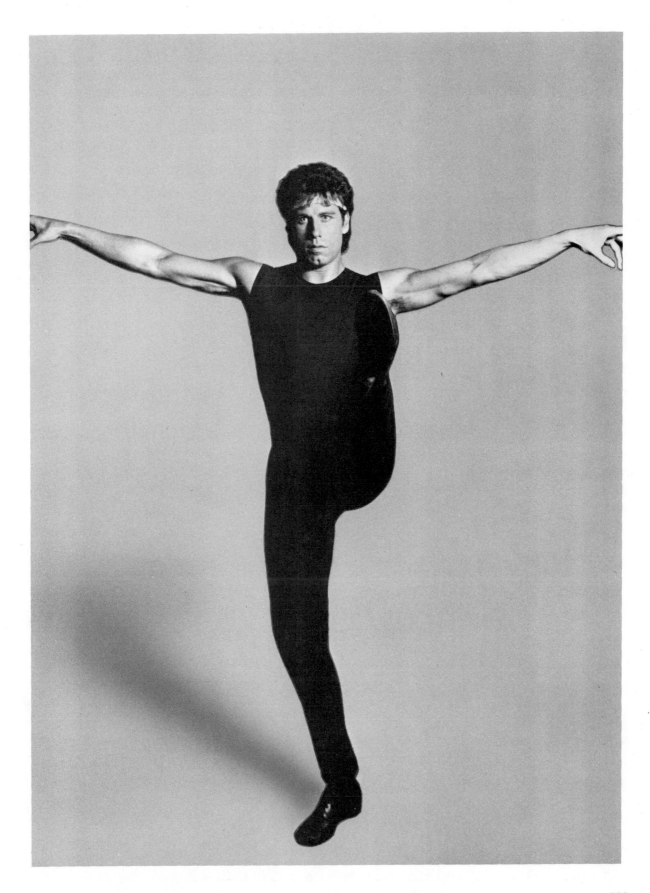

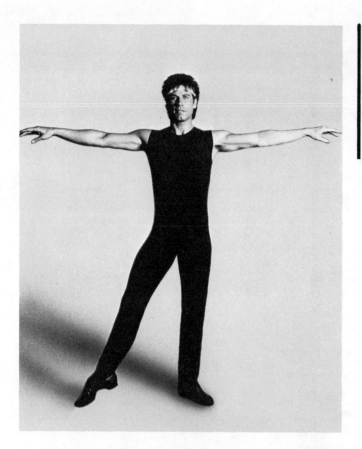

Side Kicks Description: Stand on your left leg and point your right foot to the right side. Keep your arms to the side. Begin by stepping back on your right leg behind your left in plié, then step to the side with your left leg, remaining in plié, and then step front with your right leg and kick your left leg out to the side, just slightly in front of your body, straightening your right leg.

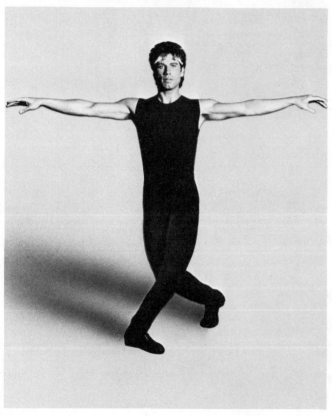

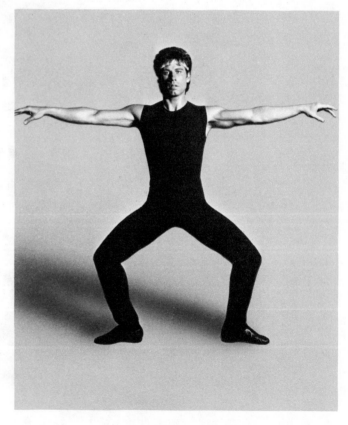

This is a three-step preparation to kick. You will go on to the next side by taking the leg you just kicked back down behind your right leg. Then step to the side with your right leg, step front with your left leg and kick your right leg to the side.

Repetitions: Each step is 1 count and the kick is the fourth count. Do a total of four kicks on each leg.

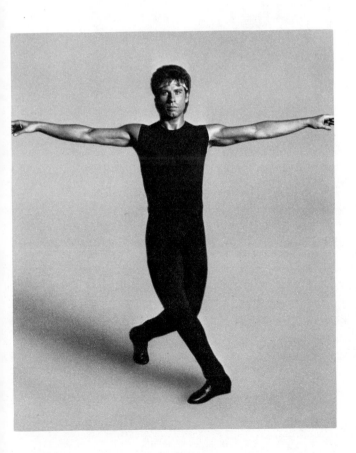
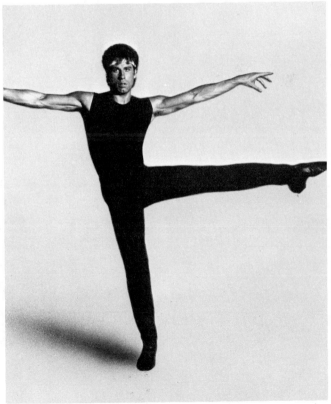

Back Kicks Description: Bring back the chair for support. Hold the chair with both hands. Stand on your left leg and place your right leg behind you with the foot pointed. Kick your right leg up as high behind you as you can and return it to the pointed position.

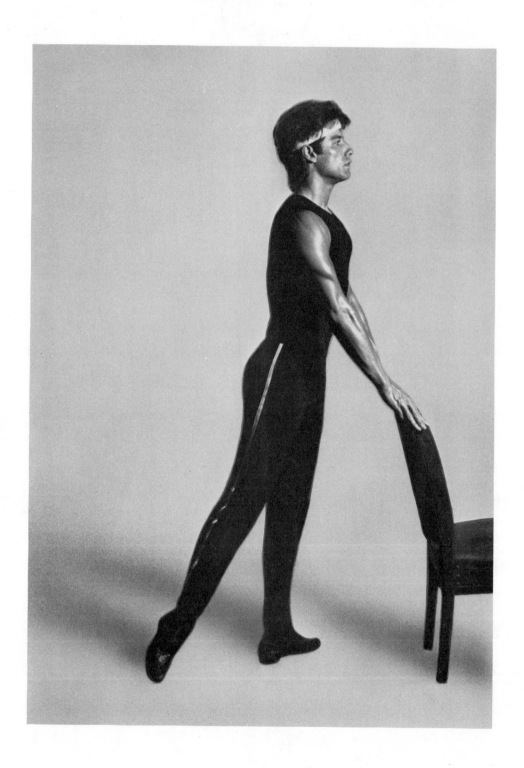

Repetitions: *Use 1 count to kick and 1 count to place the foot back on the floor. Do four kicks on the right leg. Then change your stance and kick your left leg four times.*
Remove the chair.

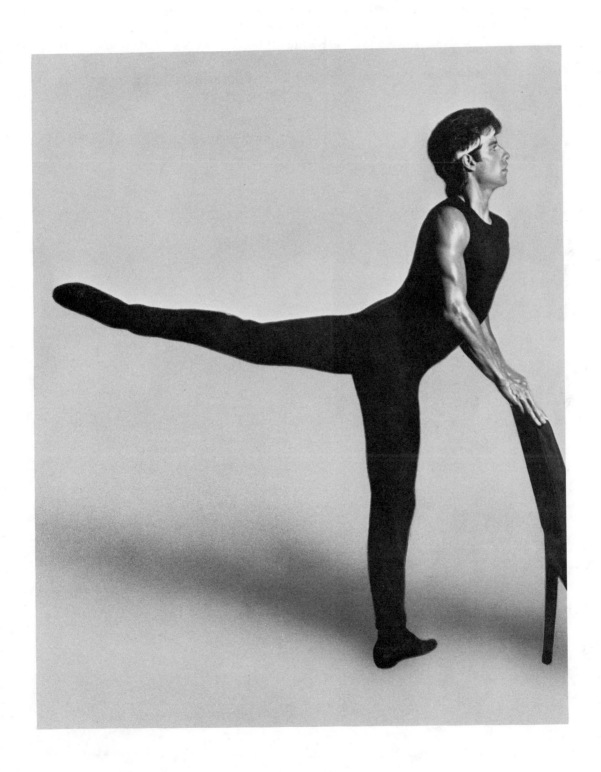

JUMPS

This exercise works your legs, ankles, feet and your heart.

Description: Start with your feet tight together and parallel. Place your arms down by your sides. Do three knee bends or demi-pliés in a bouncing fashion, and jump straight up in the air after the last one. Straighten your legs and point your feet. When you land, bend your knees. Work to keep your back as straight as possible so it is your legs doing the work and not your back.

Repetitions: Do the three bends and jump a total of four times. Rest 16 counts and repeat.

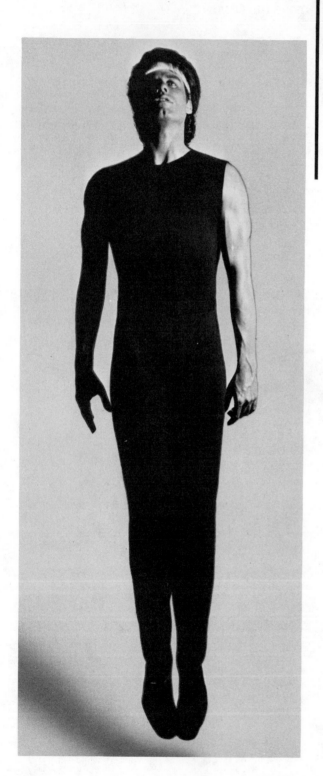

Standing Stretch Finish

INTERMEDIATE
APPROXIMATELY SIX MINUTES

PLIÉS

Same as the beginners (page 98–100).

CALF RISES

*Do the complete beginners version (page 100), then add to it the following **Straight-Leg Rises.***

Description: Keeping your feet together, raise and lower your body, as in the beginners Calf Rises, but without the plié in between. You will rise up on the balls of the feet and then descend until your feet are flat on the floor.

Repetitions: Do eight rises. On the eighth repetition, stay up in the raised position and hold for 8 counts while you let go of the chair and balance. Then repeat.

KICKS

Do the front, side, and back kicks as described in the beginners stretch (pages 102–107). This time do a total of six kicks on each leg.

JUMPS

Do the jumps as described in the beginners section (page 108), with a variation on the count. This time do only two bends and jump twice instead of once. Take 1 count for each movement. Repeat this four times for a total of eight jumps. Rest for 16 counts and repeat.

Standing Stretch Finish

ADVANCED
APPROXIMATELY EIGHT MINUTES

The advanced version is done without the use of the chair. You will now have to rely on your own strength, coordination, and balance to execute the movements.

PLIÉS

Do the same number that you did in the beginners version (page 98), but now incorporate arm movements.

Description: Start the demi-plié with your arms down by your sides. As you bend your knees, open your arms away from your body about twelve inches and bring them back down to your sides as you straighten your legs. On the grand pliés, extend your arms to the side in line with your shoulders to help maintain your balance, and bring them back to your body as you straighten.

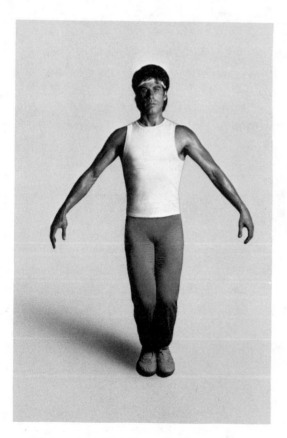

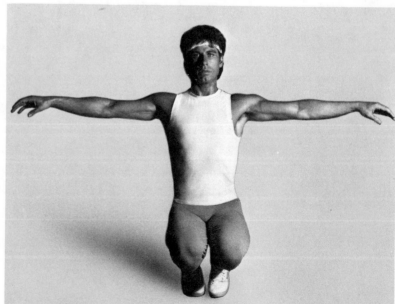

Repetitions: Do a set of demi- and grand pliés with feet parallel, then do a set in first position (feet and knees turned out). Take 2 counts to bend and 2 counts to come up. Then repeat the exercises, taking 4 counts to go down and 4 counts to come up.

When working without the chair, you need to concentrate more intensely on making your legs bend smoothly without any sudden jerky motions. Also, work to keep your back in a straight, upright position. Remember to put that imaginary girdle around your stomach.

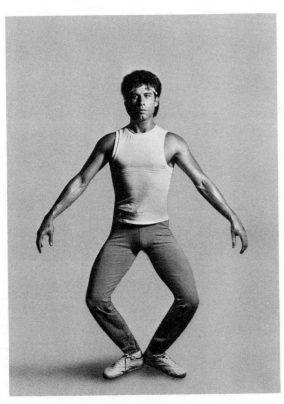

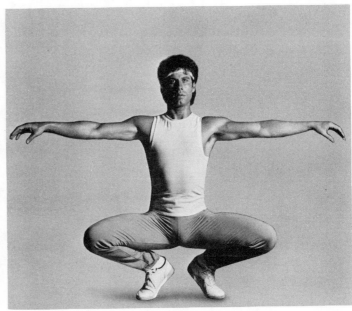

CALF RISES

Do these and the Straight-Leg Rises as described in the Intermediate section (page 109), but without the chair. Stretch your arms to the side for balance.

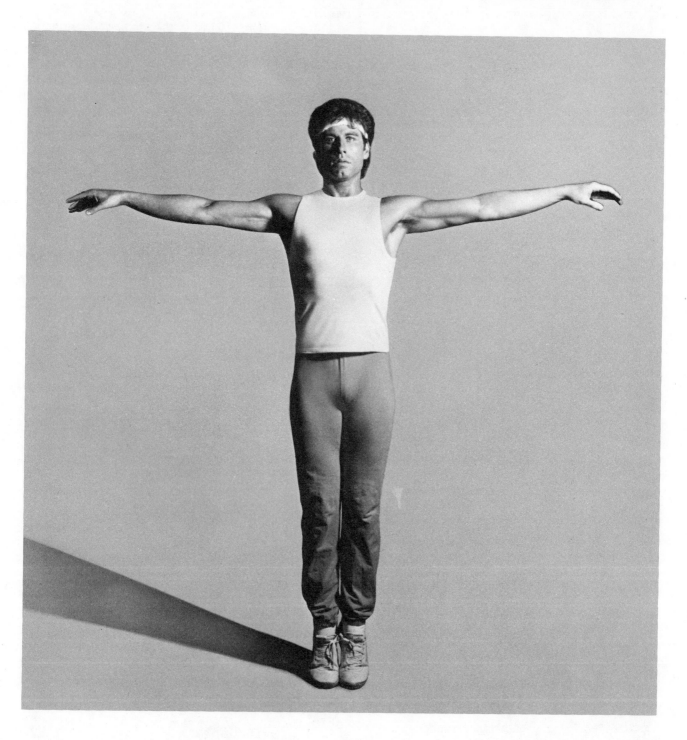

KICKS

Increase the kicks (pages 102–107) to eight repetitions on each leg.

JUMPS

*Do all the intermediate jumps (page 109) and then add these **Open Side Jumps.***

Description: *Use the three-bend preparation and jump, as in the beginners exercise (page 108). This time, as you jump, open your legs out to the side (about three feet apart) and bring them back together when you land. Make sure you bend your knees when you land. Bending your knees is what cushions your landing so you don't jar your back or knees.*

Repetitions: *Do four jumps. Rest for 16 counts and repeat.*

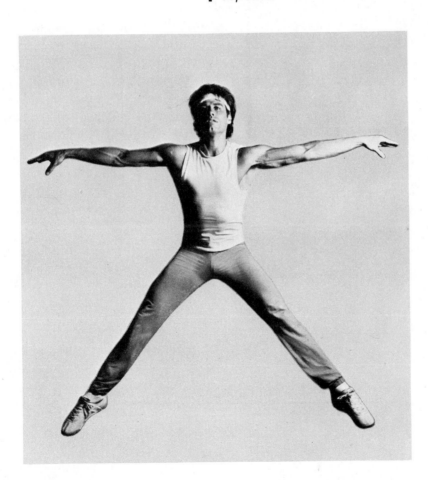

Partner Stretch

APPROXIMATELY TEN MINUTES
SUGGESTED FOR
INTERMEDIATE
AND ADVANCED
WORKOUTS ONLY.

Demonstrated here with Marilu Henner—Marilu follows the program described in my book—is a ten-minute continuous stretch routine. It can be done in addition to the regular Standing Stretch and Floor Stretch, or you can substitute it for one of these once or twice a week.

You will have to do this a few times before you can memorize the routine. When you have memorized it, begin to dance it. Make it flow smoothly from one exercise to the next. Pay particular attention to the transitions, so you progress smoothly without stopping from one exercise to the next. Each transition should take 8 counts to execute. However, when first learning the movements, take all the time you need to execute them correctly.

ARM RESISTANCE

Great as an overall arm stretch, and for the shoulder area.

Starting Position: Both you and your partner face the same direction, with the man in back of the woman. Stand close together so there is no space between you. Place your feet in a parallel position, with the woman's slightly inside the man's. Place your arms down to your sides with the woman's hands resting on top of the man's.

Description: The man begins by lifting his arm sideways above head level. The woman presses down on his arms while he does this to provide strong resistance to his movement. The man stops his arms when he gets them to the "V" position above his head.

Then, to lower them, the woman presses her arms back down to her sides while the man resists, so she has to work to bring her arms down.

Repetitions: Take 8 counts to go up and 8 counts to come down. Do this twice in 8 counts and then twice using only 4 counts.

When doing this exercise, keep your stomach muscles pulled up and your shoulders down. The amount of pressure supplied by each partner should provide only enough resistance so you feel the arm and back muscles work. The resistance should not keep your partner from completing the movement.

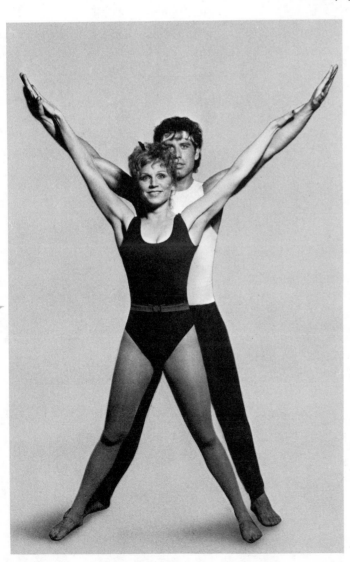

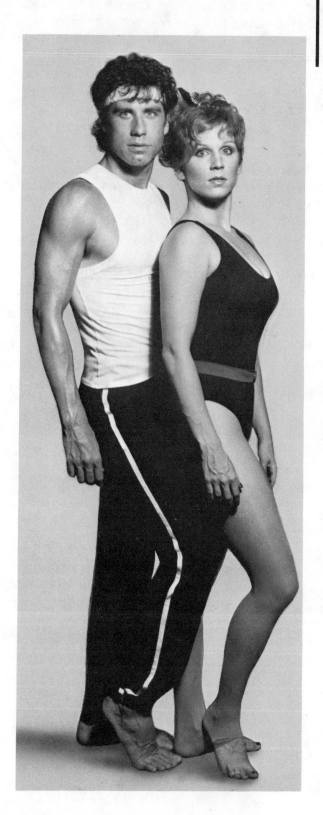

Transition: With the man still in back of the woman, each of you bring your right leg next to your left leg. Then both of you slide your right foot forward about two and a half feet. The right foot should be slightly turned out, at about 45 degrees. Your legs should be straight and your arms straight out to the sides.

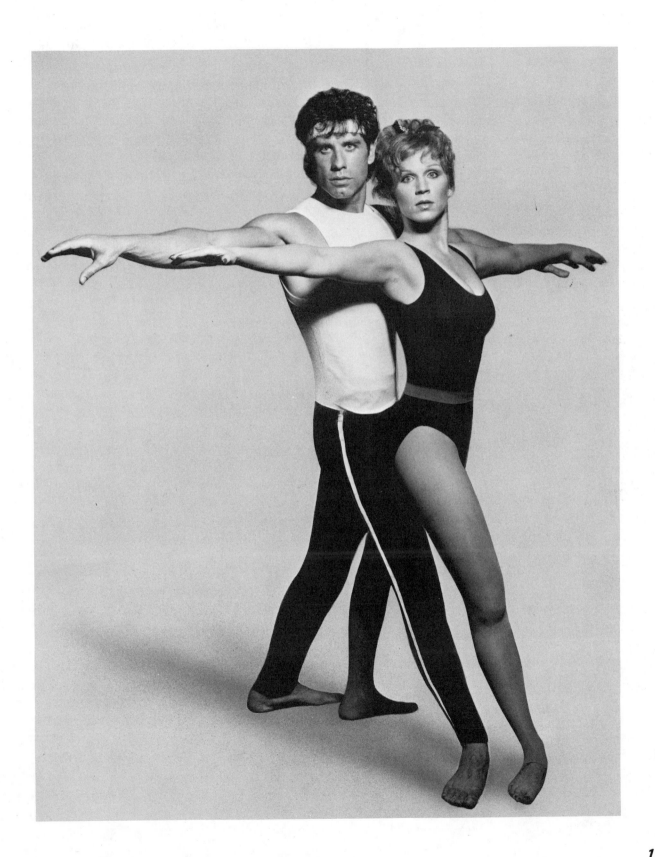

FRONT LUNGES

This works the thighs and develops overall leg strength. In addition, it develops side and front stretch.

Description: Begin together by bending your right leg into a lunge position. Make sure that your knee is in direct alignment with your foot, and keep your heels down on the floor. After you have reached the full lunge position, straighten up.

Repetitions: Do two lunges, using 4 counts to bend and 4 counts to straighten.

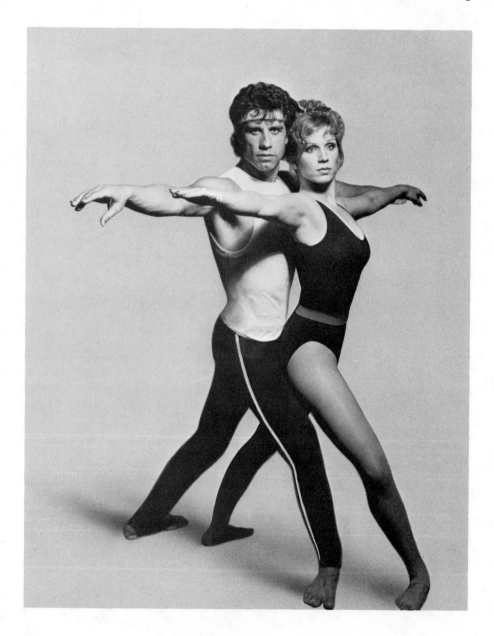

Description: Holding the straight-leg position, bend your upper body sideways to the right, rounding your arms, and then return your torso to the upright position. Repeat on the other side.

To change legs, bring your right leg back to your left and then slide your left foot forward. Repeat the exercise on your left leg.

Repetitions: Take 4 counts to bend your upper body sideways to the right, and 4 counts to come back to center. Then bend your upper body to the left for 4 counts and take 4 counts to come back to center. Do the exercise twice in both directions.

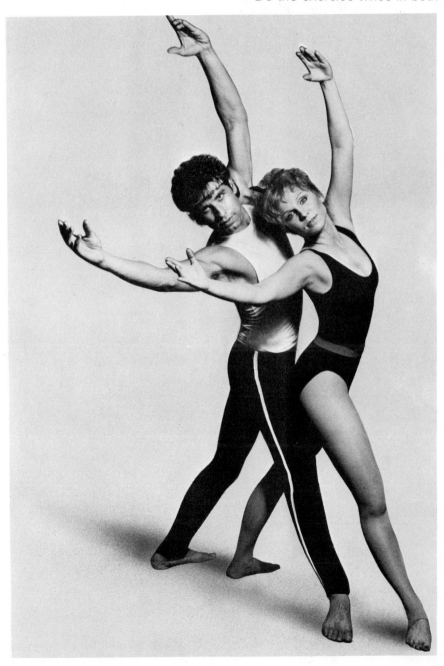

Transition: After completing the lunge exercise on your left leg, the woman should step forward, bringing her legs together, and turn to face the man. The man should bring his left foot back next to his right and place his feet together. You are now facing each other with your legs together. Reach out and take hold of each other's wrists. The palms of the man's hands should be facing up. The woman's should be facing down. Your legs should be straight. Lean away from each other, keeping your body straight, as though you were on a slant board. You will be leaning away from each other at about a 30-degree angle.

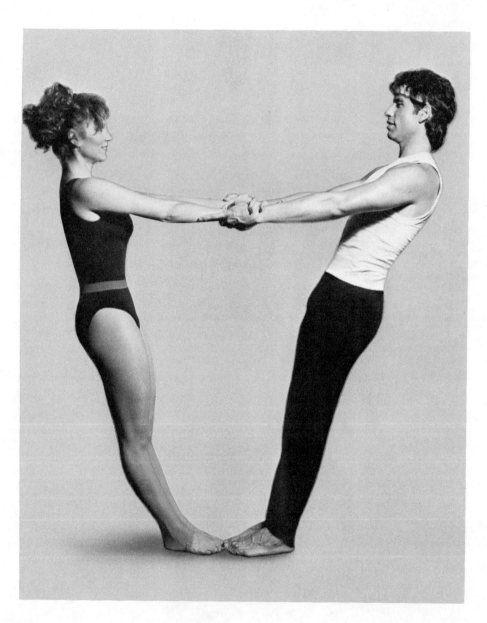

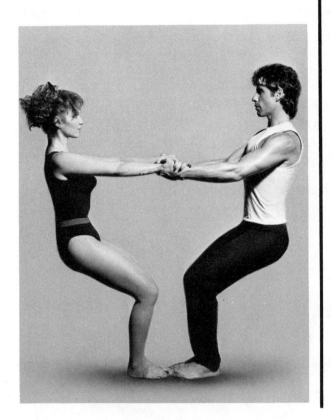

MIRROR-IMAGE PLIÉS

These are great for upper body strength as well as for the legs.

Description: Do two demi-pliés. Keep hold of each other's wrists and keep your arms straight. When doing the demi-pliés, it should feel as if you are sitting on a chair. Then do two grand pliés. Here you will continue down past the halfway point until you are almost sitting on the floor.

Repetitions: Take 4 counts down for the demi-plié, and 4 counts to come up. Take 8 counts down for the grand plié and 8 counts to come up. During the exercise maintain the pull-away resistance.

This exercise may take some practice until you get the right amount of tension on your arms so one of you doesn't fall off balance.

Transition: After the grand pliés above, do one more plié. This time go all the way down and sit on the floor. Keep hold of each other's hands. Place the soles of your feet against your partner's and straighten your legs so you slide away from each other. If you haven't the stretch in your legs to straighten them all the way, keep them slightly bent.

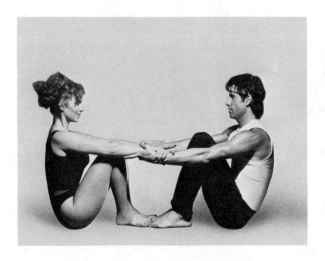

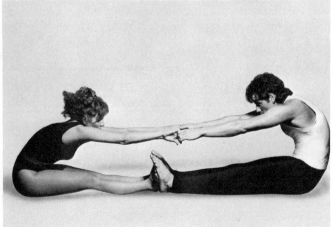

FORWARD STRETCH

This stretches your hamstrings and works the back muscles.

Description: *Both start with backs as straight as possible. The man pulls backward as the woman stretches forward. This is a slow stretch. Be careful not to pull back too hard or in a jerky fashion or you might overstretch your partner's hamstrings. Return to a center position, backs as straight as possible. Then the woman pulls back, stretching the man forward. Return to the center position.*

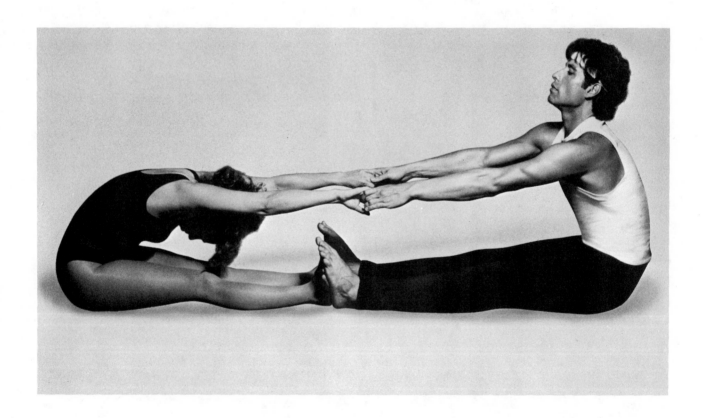

Repetitions: Use 8 slow counts for the man to pull back, and 8 counts to come to the center position. Then use 8 counts for the woman to pull back, and 8 counts to come to center. Then repeat.

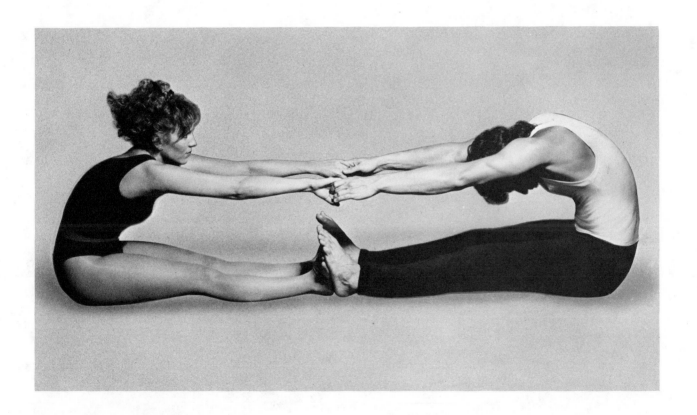

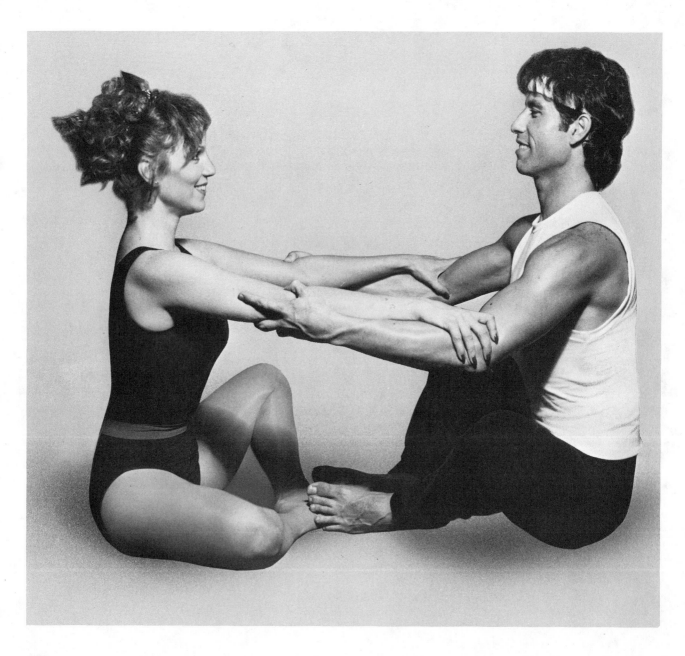

MIRROR LOTUS

This exercise works your hips, inside thighs, and back.

Description: Do the same movement you did for the Forward Stretch. Start with your backs straight.

Repetitions: The man will lean back for 8 counts and then return to an upright position for 8 counts. Then the woman leans back. Repeat.

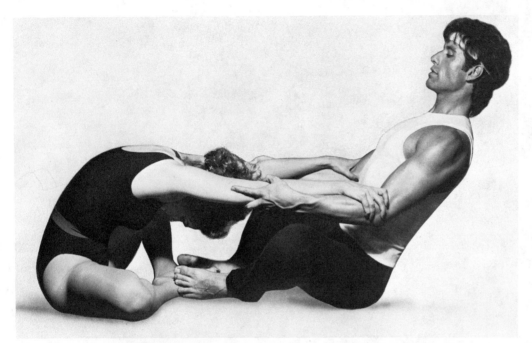

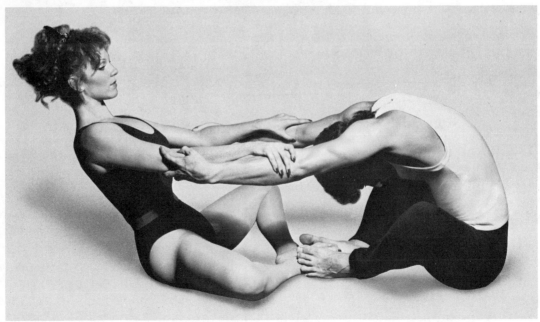

Transition: Slide your grip back to your wrists and open your legs to the sides. Let your feet touch and remain braced against each other as you open your legs as wide as your stretch will allow. Straighten your back as much as you can.

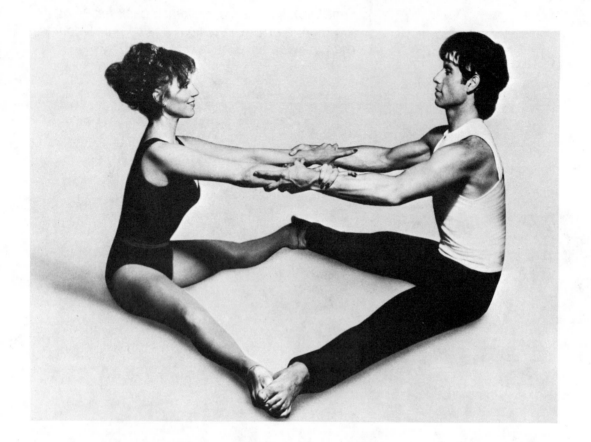

OPEN SPLIT—MIRROR IMAGE

This stretches your inner thighs and your hamstrings.

Description: As you mirror each other's movement, the man will lean back as the woman stretches forward. The man should pull gently so his partner stretches forward a little more than she normally can. It's up to the woman to tell her partner how far she can go. Return to the upright position, and then the woman leans back, stretching the man. During the exercise, keep your feet pointed.

Repetitions: Take 8 counts for the man to lean back as the woman stretches forward. Then 8 counts to come up to an upright position. Use the same counts while the woman leans back and comes up. Do these stretches smoothly. As your body stretches, you may need to take a higher grip on the arm: Instead of the wrists, try holding the elbows.

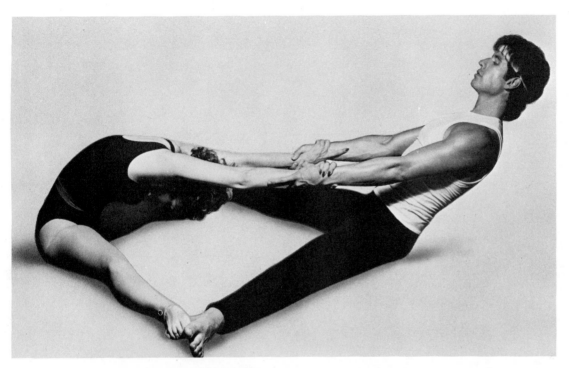

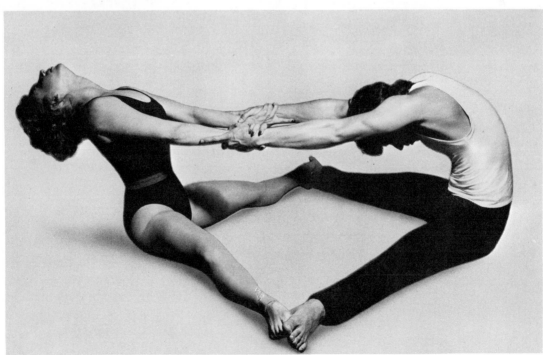

Transition: Now release your grip and lie back on the floor. Bring your legs closer together, bend your knees, and place your feet flat on the floor. The man's legs should overlap his partner's so his feet are on the outside of her hips and her feet are outside his thighs. Place your hands on your partner's feet. Apply enough pressure to keep your partner's feet on the floor during the sit-up exercise.

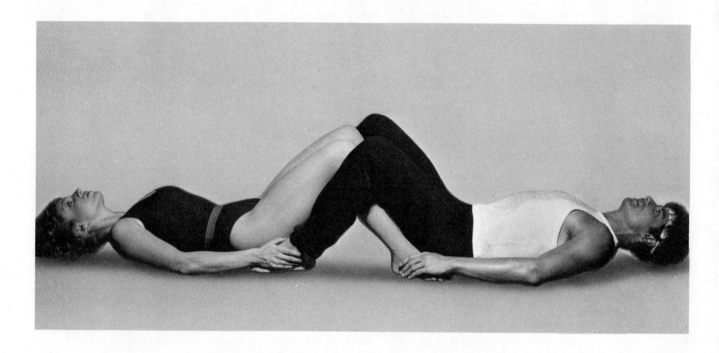

MIRROR SIT-UPS

Tightens and strengthens stomach muscles.

Description: *These are regular sit-ups, done while facing each other. Begin by lifting your shoulders and head off the floor while your back is held in a rounded contraction. Your chin should be held toward your chest as you lift up and release back to the floor. Come only halfway up in the sit-up position, just enough to feel your stomach muscles tighten and contract.*

Repetitions: *Do three sit-ups and hold the third one in the up position for two extra counts, then release down. The counts are: sit up on count 1, release down on 2, up on 3, down on 4, up on 5 (the third sit-up); hold for counts 6 and 7 as you look at each other and keep the pressure on each other's feet, and then release down on count 8. Continue without stopping for a total of four times. You may increase the number of repetitions as you need them.*

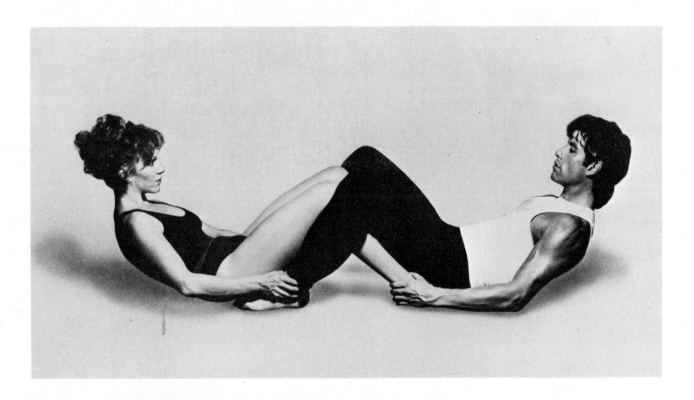

Transition: Placing your hands on the floor for support, sit up. Bend your legs in toward your body. The man should bring his feet up underneath him and get up on his knees. The woman brings her feet up under her and turns away from the man so you both are facing the same direction. Place your knees apart, about twelve to sixteen inches. The woman's feet should fit between the man's knees. Open your arms to the side.

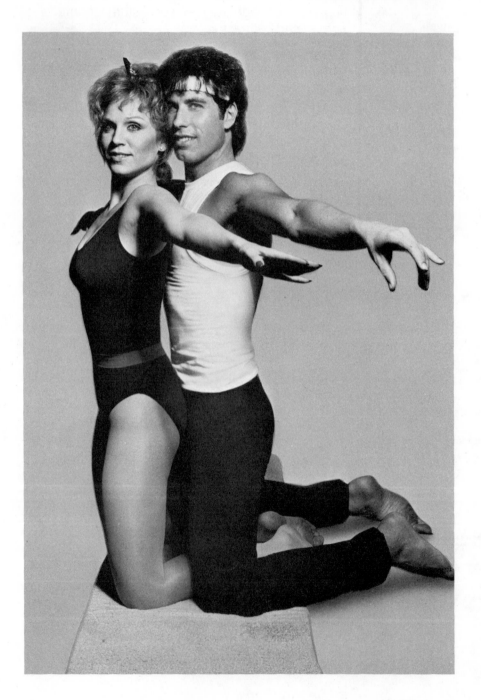

KNEE HINGES

This exercise tightens and tones the buttocks, thighs, stomach and back.

Description: In a hinge, you hold your body stiff and rigid from your knees up to your head while bending slowly back to about a 45-degree angle. The body works like a door hinge. Keep your bodies close together (the woman's back to the man's chest). Begin by slowly leaning back as the man wraps his arms around his partner. As you reach the peak of the hinge (45 degrees) the man will have completed wrapping his arms around the woman. Then unfold the arms as you both return to the upright position.

Repetitions: Use 4 counts to hinge back and 4 counts to come up. Do this a total of four times.

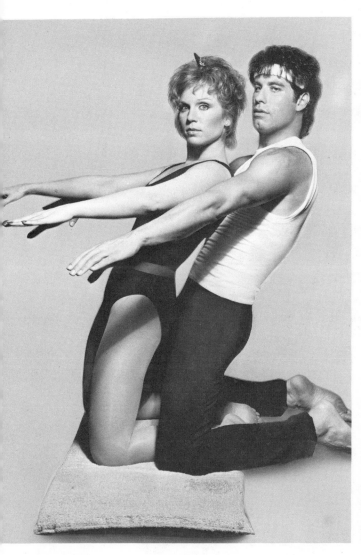
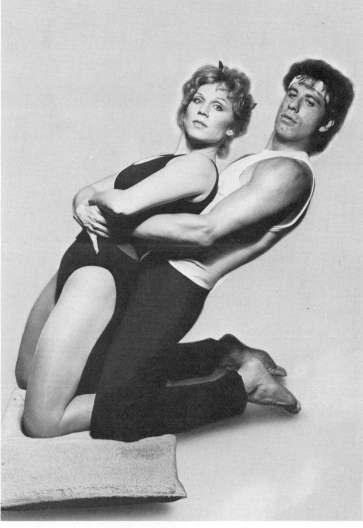

Transition: With your weight on your left knee, straighten your right leg to the side. Place your arms straight out to the side.

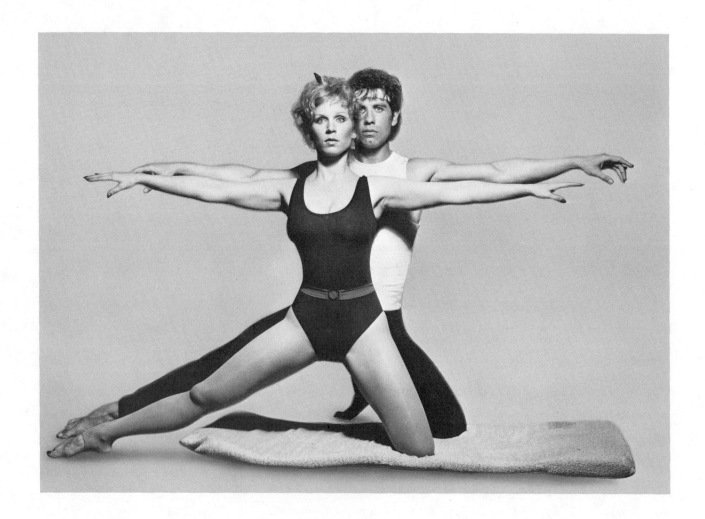

SIDE STRETCH

Description: Begin by taking your arms up above your head in a rounded oval shape, framing your face. Then lean and stretch to the right.

Repetitions: Take 4 counts to stretch to the right and 4 counts slowly to come up. Repeat. Then change sides: bring your right leg back in, kneel on it, and straighten your left leg to the side. Do the side stretch to the left twice.

Transition: The man remains in his position while the woman turns on her knees to face the man. Remain about twelve inches apart. The woman's arms are down at her sides and the man's hands are placed on the woman's shoulders, with his arms straight (see page 134).

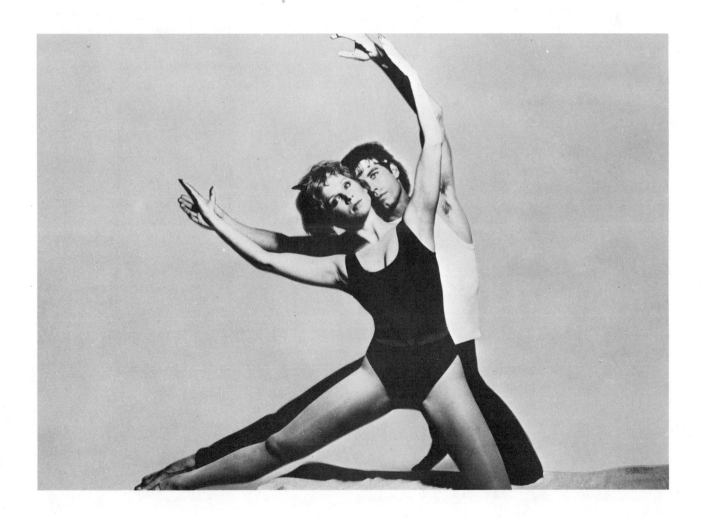

HINGE-UPS

This uses the entire body, and is great for the arms, thighs, stomach, and back.

Description: The man begins by bracing himself against the woman. Keeping his arms straight, balls of feet on the floor, he lifts his body up to straighten his legs. His body ends up in a straight line from head to toes, angled toward the woman. Then he releases down. Then the woman places her hands on her partner's shoulders as he drops his arms to his sides. The woman lifts herself up to a straight line, bracing herself on her partner, and then releases down. The kneeling partner has to hold his or her body in a locked position. This takes a certain amount of tension, which brings the whole body into play.

Repetitions: The working partner should take 4 counts to push up, 4 counts to hold the position, and 4 counts to come down slowly, taking care not to drop suddenly to the knees. Take as much care in coming down slowly as you do in going up. Then the kneeling partner takes a turn, using the same counts. Both partners repeat one more time.

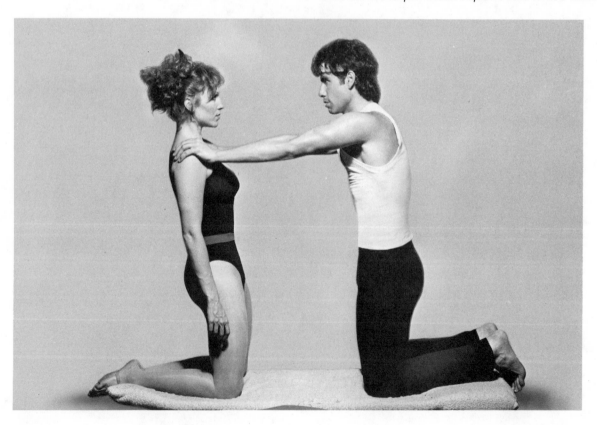

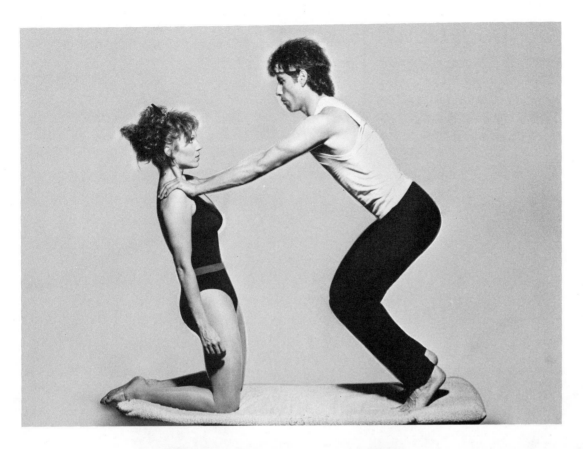

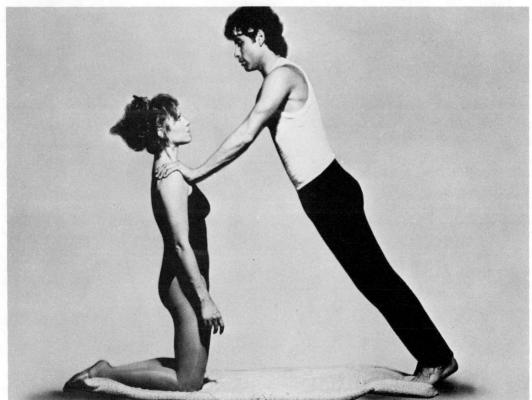

Cool-Down

*BEGINNERS,
INTERMEDIATE
AND ADVANCED
APPROXIMATELY TWO MINUTES*

Stand with your legs apart (about two feet), your feet in a parallel position, and your hands on your hips.

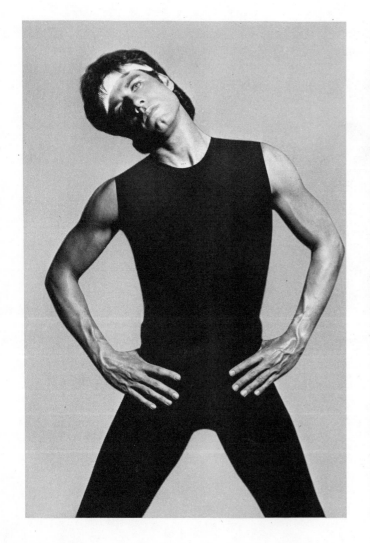

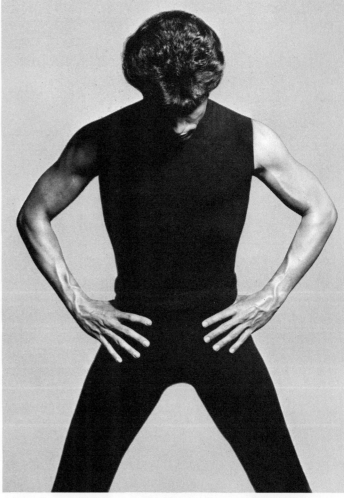

SLOW HEAD ROLLS

Description: *Start by placing your right ear close to your right shoulder. Now roll your chin to your chest and then up to the other side, bringing your left ear close to your left shoulder. Then continue the circle, lifting your chin up as you look straight up at the ceiling, then bringing your right ear toward your right shoulder.*

Repetitions: *Take a slow 8 counts to complete one circle—4 counts to bring your ear close to your shoulder, and 4 counts to complete the circle. Continue in the same direction for a total of two times, then reverse and circle twice in the other direction.*

Note: You should do these head circles slowly and in a relaxed manner. Keep your shoulders down, especially when the head is to the back.

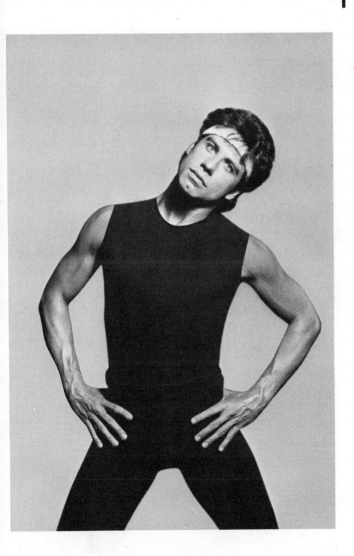
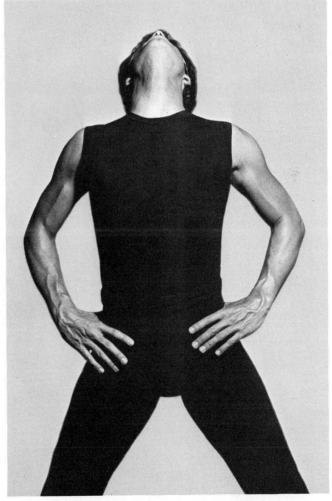

SHOULDER ROLLS

Description: Place your arms down alongside your body and begin by lifting your shoulders to your ears in a shrug position. Pull them back by bringing your shoulder blades together, and then relax your shoulders down.

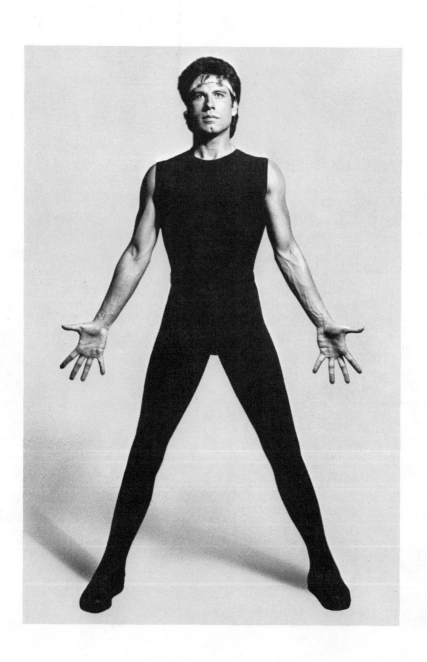

Repetitions: Take 4 counts to complete one roll. Continue in the same direction four times and then reverse the movement by lifting the shoulders, pushing them forward, and relaxing down for a total of four times.

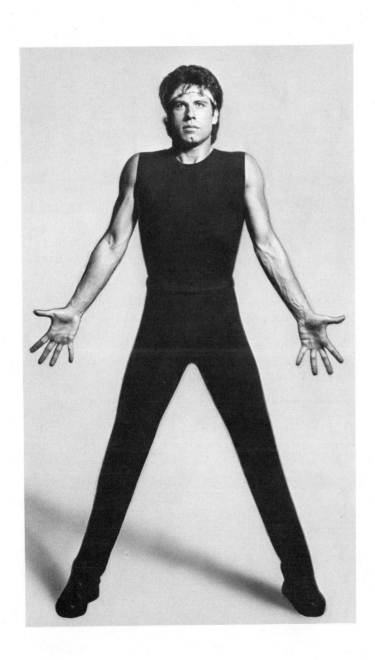

REACH AND DROP

Description: Keep your stance the same as above, but start with your arms down at your sides. Begin by placing both arms over your head and reaching up with them as high as you can. Then drop your

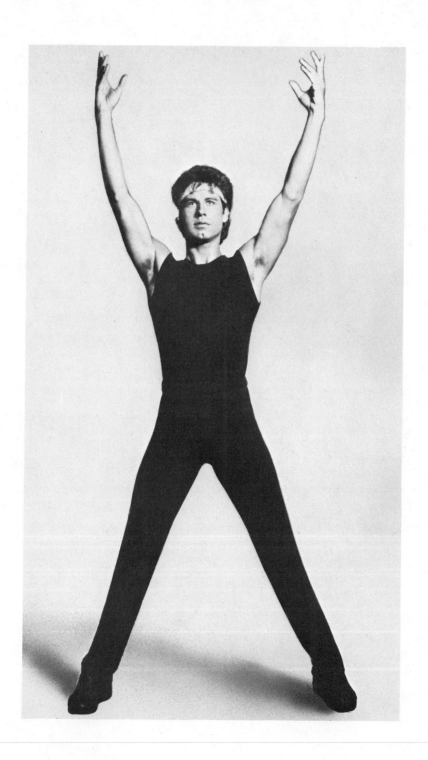

arms to your sides, bend your knees, and relax your back and head in a rounded position so you are now squatting low. Your fingertips will be just touching the floor. Hold, then roll up to the starting position.

Repetitions: Reach with arms over your head for 4 counts. Take 4 counts to descend into the squat. Hold for 4 counts, then take 4 counts to roll up to the starting position. Do the complete exercise twice. Then repeat for a third time to the squat position, from which proceed to Slow Roll-Up (page 142).

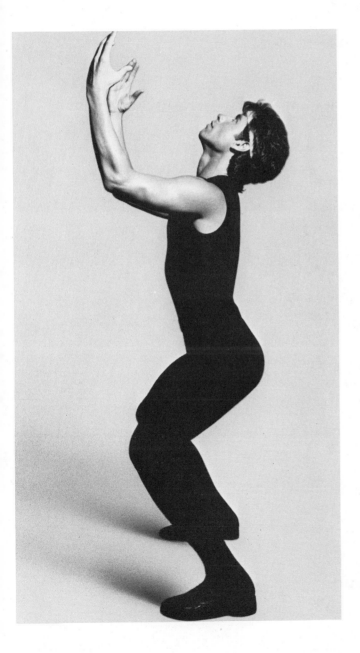
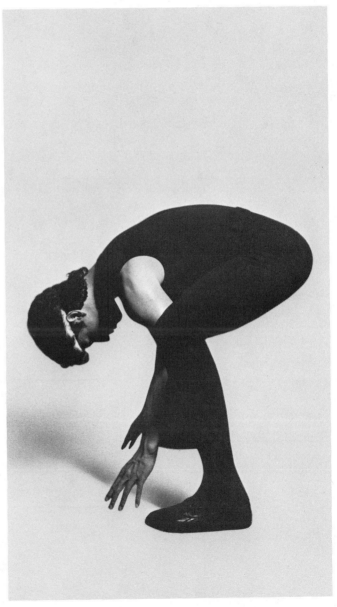

SLOW ROLL-UP

Description: After the last squat above, keep your head and back relaxed and slowly, in 16 counts, straighten your legs as you simultaneously lift your back and head to the upright position. The last thing to come up is your head, on count 16. Don't rush, take your time, and relax as you come up.

Repetitions: Do this exercise once.

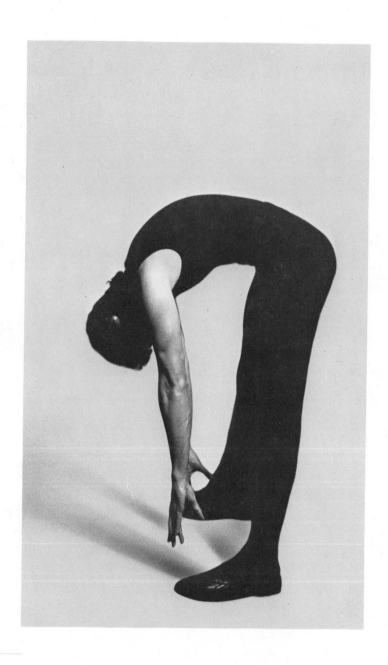

SHAKE IT OUT

Description: Bring your legs together in a more relaxed stance. Hold your right arm out to the side a little and shake out any tension that might remain. Keep your fingers relaxed and limp. Then shake your left arm in the same way. Stand on your left leg and shake out your right foot and ankle, and then reverse and shake out your left foot and ankle.

Repetitions: Take 4 counts to shake each arm, 4 counts for each foot.

DEEP BREATHING

Take a deep breath and exhale all of it. Repeat two or three times.

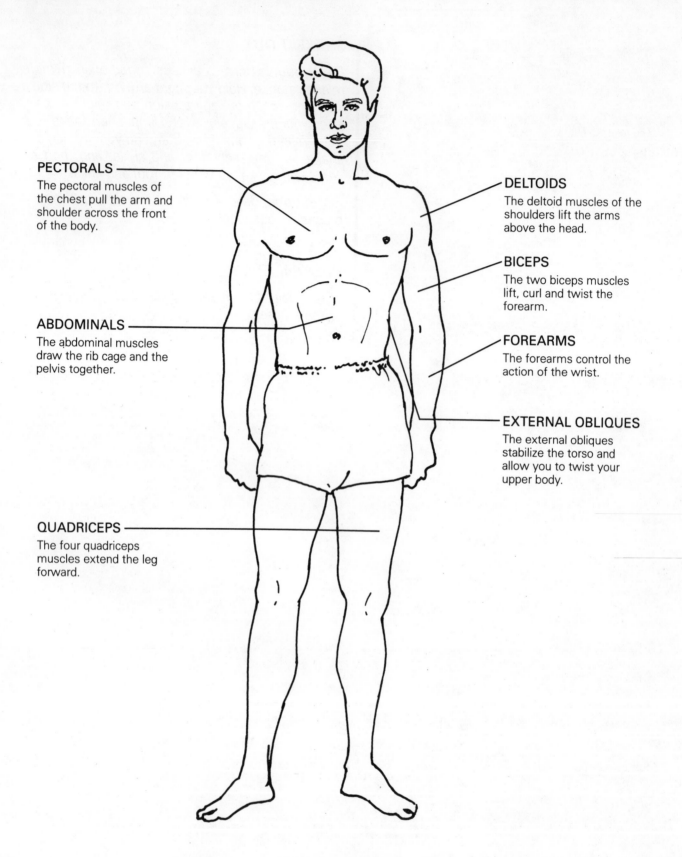

PECTORALS

The pectoral muscles of the chest pull the arm and shoulder across the front of the body.

ABDOMINALS

The abdominal muscles draw the rib cage and the pelvis together.

QUADRICEPS

The four quadriceps muscles extend the leg forward.

DELTOIDS

The deltoid muscles of the shoulders lift the arms above the head.

BICEPS

The two biceps muscles lift, curl and twist the forearm.

FOREARMS

The forearms control the action of the wrist.

EXTERNAL OBLIQUES

The external obliques stabilize the torso and allow you to twist your upper body.

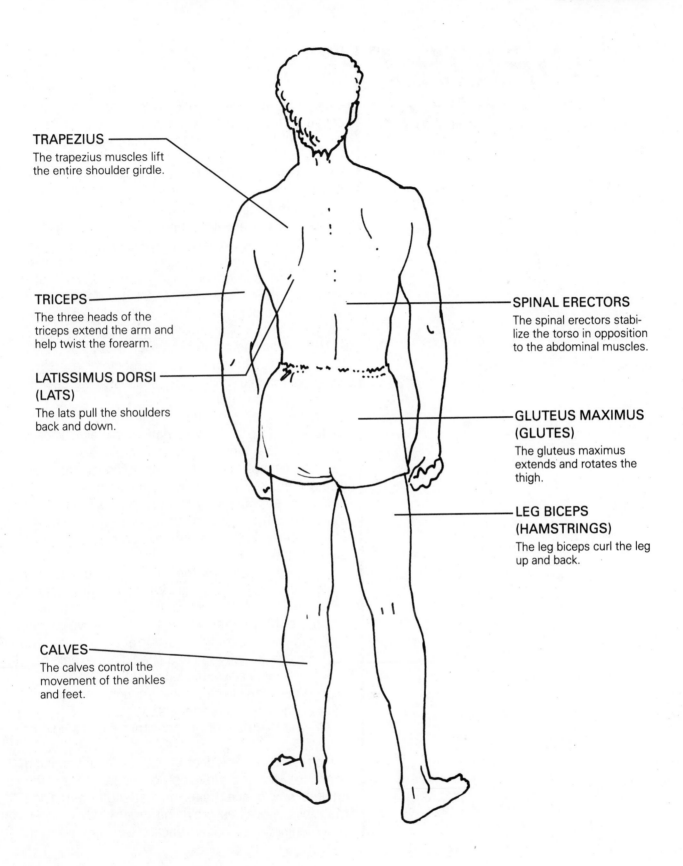

TRAPEZIUS
The trapezius muscles lift the entire shoulder girdle.

TRICEPS
The three heads of the triceps extend the arm and help twist the forearm.

LATISSIMUS DORSI (LATS)
The lats pull the shoulders back and down.

SPINAL ERECTORS
The spinal erectors stabilize the torso in opposition to the abdominal muscles.

GLUTEUS MAXIMUS (GLUTES)
The gluteus maximus extends and rotates the thigh.

LEG BICEPS (HAMSTRINGS)
The leg biceps curl the leg up and back.

CALVES
The calves control the movement of the ankles and feet.

WEIGHT TRAINING

When getting in shape for *Staying Alive* I worked out every day, and though the pain of the first few weeks had me sweating and swearing, I was so excited by the results that I've become a complete convert. Now I can't imagine *not* working out. I have used both Universal and Paramount equipment and both work extremely well in conjunction with various free weights. And I try to spread the good word about working out wherever I go. Which is one reason I'm writing this book.

Personally, I always found the exercises for the legs, chest, and biceps relatively easy. Exercising these muscles seemed natural. The shoulder exercises were something else. These *hurt!* But I wanted better shoulders—and I got better shoulders. And that's the point. You really *can* make yourself over. As for the stomach, you can't burn it enough. Make sure you exercise it *every day.* And a final word to the women—the pectoral exercises really *can* make you more shapely. I've seen it happen with my friends!

The key to progressive weight training is training to failure. This means selecting a weight heavy enough so that when you complete the last rep of a set, you cannot do another repetition of the exercise. When you have trained to the point where the final repetitions are easy to perform, it is time to add more weight. When this is true of all the exercises you are performing, it is time to advance to the next stage of the program.

Try to train with a partner. Training with a partner of your own level and ability will help your progress tremendously. Not only is the extra enthusiasm helpful, but a partner will help spot the weight for you, and will help watch your form.

There are times when you should not exercise.

1. When you are extremely tired.

2. When you do not have enough time to perform all the exercises adequately.

3. When you are ill or recovering from a cold or injury.

I have not included progressive weight training exercises for leg development because of the unique way dance trains and strengthens all leg muscles, as well as providing great cardiovascular conditioning. As you advance, you may want to

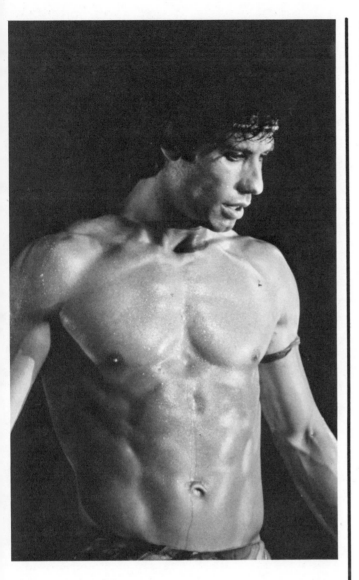

supplement the dance program with weight training exercises. These might include leg press, leg extension, leg curl, and calf raise exercises.

Here briefly are some general principles to keep in mind when doing the weight training. I hope they help you as much as they did me.

1. Do the stretch and warm-up exercises before beginning each weight training session. Cool down after each training session (see page 15).
2. Begin your exercise program by starting with your hardest or least-liked exercise.
3. Isolate the muscle group you are using and concentrate on that group throughout the exercise.
4. Vary your exercises and change your order of exercise periodically so you do not fall into training ruts.
5. Conclude each exercise by tensing the specific muscle group that you have been exercising. These tension exercises will pump more blood into the particular muscle.
6. If you find that your arms are doing most of the work, try doing your arm exercises first. This routine will pre-exhaust your smaller muscle groups, forcing you to isolate the larger muscles.
7. Breathe throughout each exercise. Inhale through your nose and exhale through your mouth. Exhale when pushing or pulling the weight or at the point of maximum exertion; inhale when returning to starting position.
   Please note: Individuals who have sinus or nose-related problems should inhale and exhale through their mouths.
8. Take small sips of water throughout the training period. Do not drink a large amount of water at one time. Do not drink extremely cold or hot water. Anything extremely hot or cold may cause cramping or abdominal discomfort.
9. Move slowly when getting into or out of an exercise position. Use your hands to push yourself up from a sitting to a standing position.
10. Never lift anything from the floor without bending your knees. In general, always have a small bend in your arms and legs.

11. As a rule, always lower weight more slowly than you raise it.
12. If possible, watch yourself in a mirror during all exercises. Watch your form and make sure you are pulling and pushing evenly.
13. Fix your eyes on a particular spot so you can look straight ahead when doing all exercises.
14. If you ever feel dizzy, stop the exercise, lie down, and raise your feet slightly.
15. Always wear tennis or running shoes while training.
16. The suggested time for each program is only an approximation. Use it as a suggested target only.

You will need the following equipment for the weight training program:

1. Ankle weights
   2½ pounds
   5 pounds
2. Dumbbells
   sets of 5, 10, 15, and 20 pounds
3. Block of wood, four-by-four,
   18 inches long (to make incline bench)
4. Flat bench
5. Universal or similar type of multiple-station equipment.

Beginner Program

*25 MINUTES
60 SECONDS BETWEEN SETS
3 DAYS PER WEEK*

Abdominals

CRUNCH

*1 set
20 repetitions*

The Crunch is a great exercise that develops the upper abdominal muscles. Lie on the floor with your calves pressed against the bench. Your back and buttocks should be resting on the floor. Position your hands behind your neck or crossed on your chest. Keep your knees as close together as possible throughout the exercise.

This is a short-range movement exercise. Begin the movement by raising your hips slightly off the floor, then raise your shoulders off the floor and push your elbows toward your upper legs. Lower toward the starting position by letting the back of your shoulders touch the floor before beginning the next repetition.

Exhale as you crunch forward. Inhale as you return to the starting position.

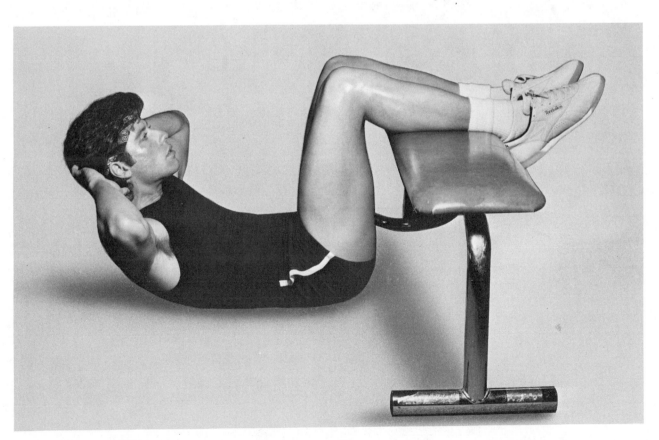

FLOOR FLEXOR

1 set
20 repetitions

Flexors strengthen the lower stomach muscles.
Lie down on your back with your palms face down underneath your buttocks, legs straight with feet flexed and raised approximately six inches off the floor. Begin the exercise by raising your knees together so that the tops of your knees are above your upper stomach. Then straighten your legs out, about six inches off the floor, keeping your knees straight. Use a moderately fast speed.
Exhale as your knees are raised toward your stomach and inhale as you stretch your legs straight.

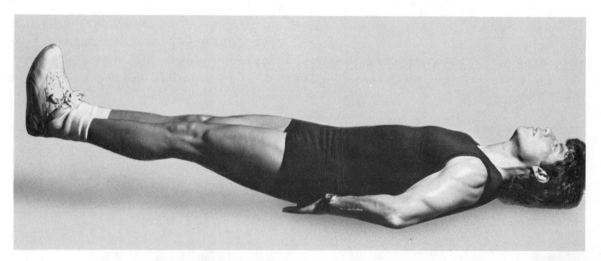

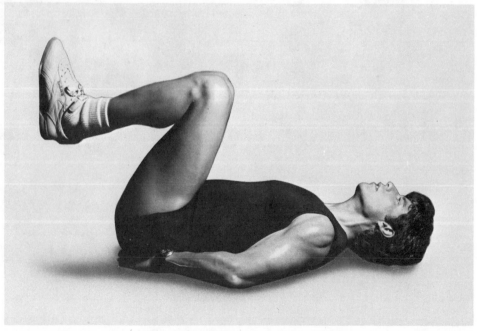

ABDOMINAL CROSS-OVERS

1 set
50 repetitions

The Abdominal Cross-Over is a unique exercise designed to tone the oblique or side muscles of the stomach. It's one of my favorite exercises—I do it all the time! Do this exercise in a standing position. Spread your feet approximately eighteen inches apart, or a little more than shoulder-width apart.

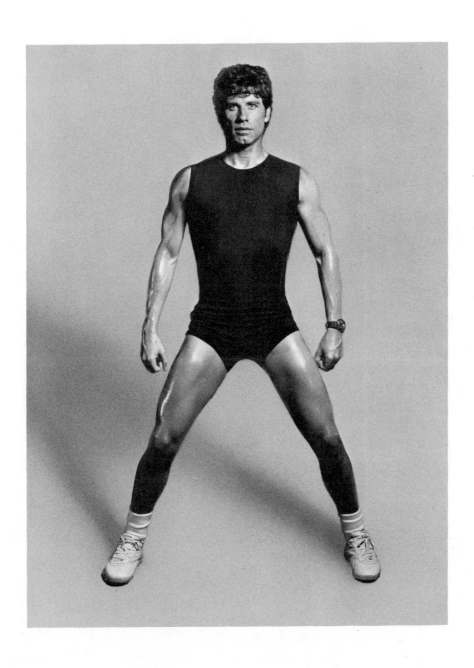

(Exercise continued on next page.)

Keeping your knees bent, stretch your right arm to the left above the top of your head as your left arm stretches across your lower stomach. This starting position is considered one count of the exercise. Rapidly reverse the position, so that your left arm is above your head and your right arm crosses your lower stomach. Both arms will swing through a semi-circular motion. This completes the second repetition of this exercise.

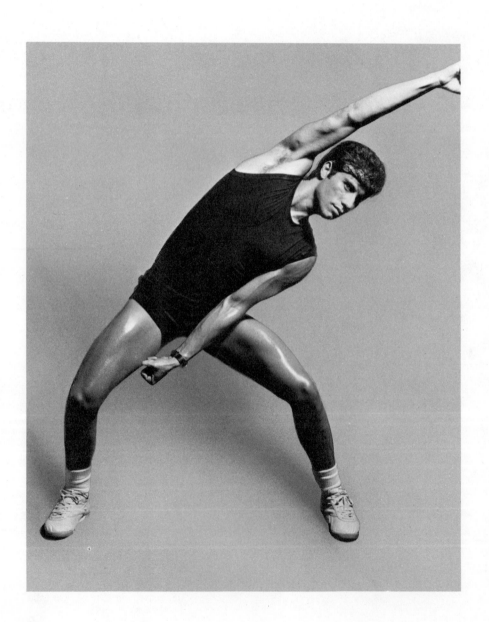

This is a rapid stretch and contraction movement for the outer part of your stomach muscle. While one side is stretched, the other side is contracted. As you improve, extend your top arm higher for added stretch. If you desire more contraction, lower the top arm so that it is closer to the top of your head.

Exhale when your arm is in an up position, inhale as you change sides.

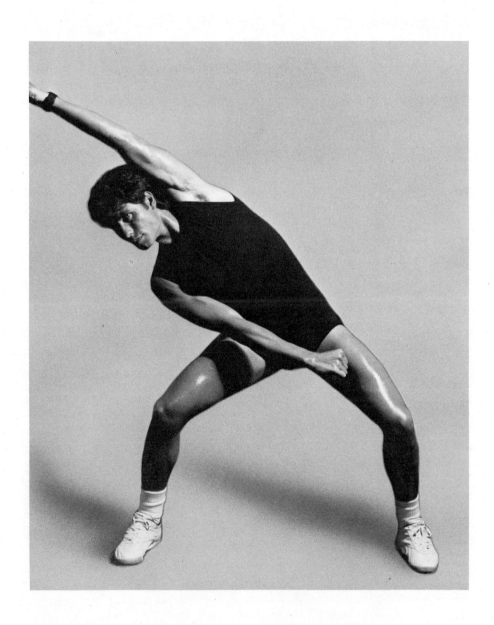

Chest

PULL-OVERS

1 set
15 repetitions

Pull-Overs will expand the rib cage and strengthen the entire upper body. Do this exercise with a five- or ten-pound weight. Use the flat bench for this exercise.

Lie on the bench on your back, head extended over the edge, heels flat on the bench with knees bent. Grip the dumbbell with your palms against the inside of the weight. With arms extended toward the ceiling, begin by slowly lowering the weight until your hands are below your head. Your arms will bend as you reach the low position. Raise the weight and progressively straighten your arms as you pull the dumbbell over your head to the starting position.

Inhale as you lower the weight. Exhale fully as you return to the starting position.

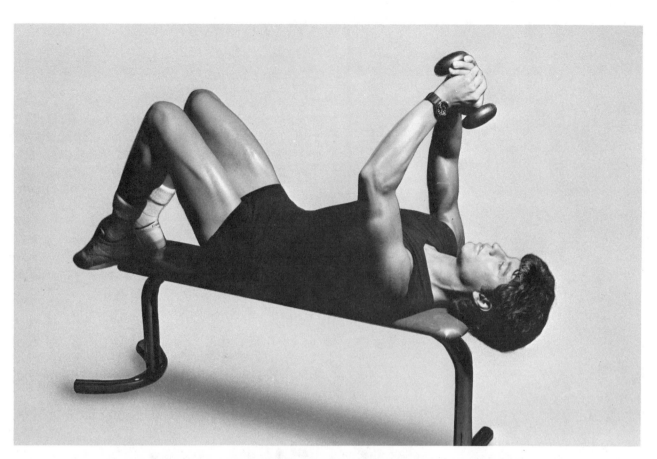

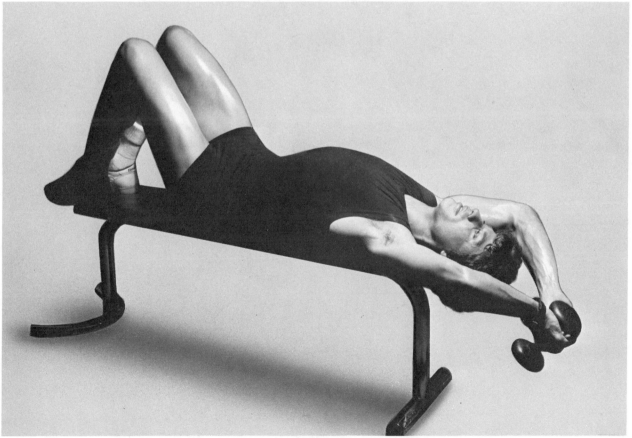

MODIFIED PUSH-UPS

1 set
15 repetitions

Push-ups remain one of the best ways to strengthen the chest muscles. A modified position is a good way to start. The exercise is demonstrated below by my friend and trainer Dan Isaacson.

Position yourself with hands and knees on the floor. Your hands should be positioned underneath your shoulders. Slowly lower your upper body until your nose almost touches the floor. Push your upper body back to the starting position, squeezing your chest muscles together at the top of the exercise.

Inhale as you move downward toward the floor, exhale as you push up from the floor.

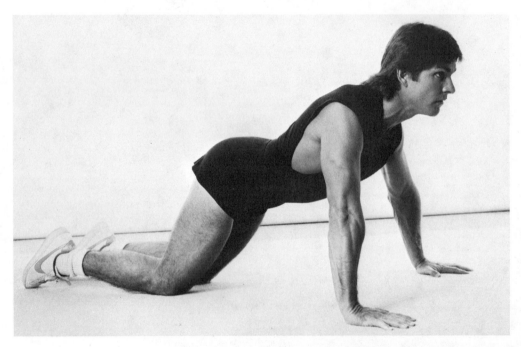

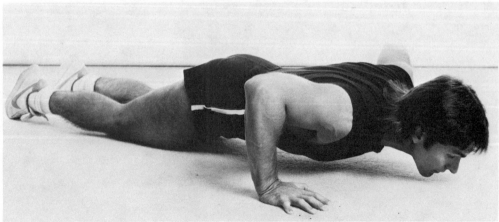

Back

DUMBBELL DEAD LIFT

1 set
15 repetitions

This is a great exercise for strengthening the spinal erector muscles, which protect the lower part of your spine, and stretching the back of the legs. Use the five-pound dumbbells for this exercise. Hold them in front of you so that the ends of each dumbbell touch each other. Place your feet about twelve inches apart. I'm a dancer and used to keeping my legs straight when I exercise, but I recommend that most of you bend your legs slightly when lifting a weight.

As if you were doing a simple toe touch, lower your arms toward the floor while keeping your back straight and shoulders rolled back. When you are as low as possible, pause for a count of two and then slowly return to your standing position.

Inhale as you lower yourself and exhale as you rise to the starting position.

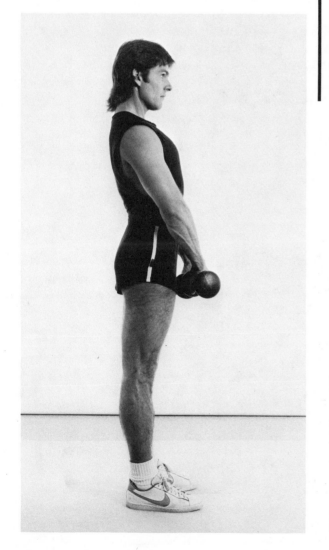

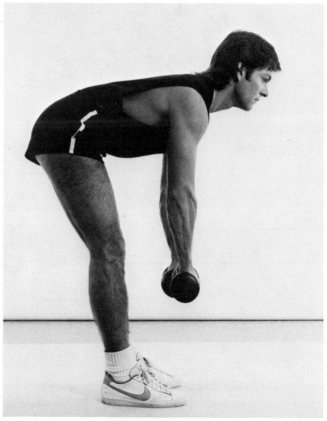

ROWING

1 set
15 repetitions

When properly executed, rowing is an excellent exercise for the large muscle of your back, the latissimus dorsi muscle or, more commonly, the "lats."

Use the five- or ten-pound dumbbells for this exercise. Hold the dumbbells at your sides. Position your feet so they are about six inches apart and slightly bend your knees. With your back straight, bend over with your upper body as parallel to the floor as possible.

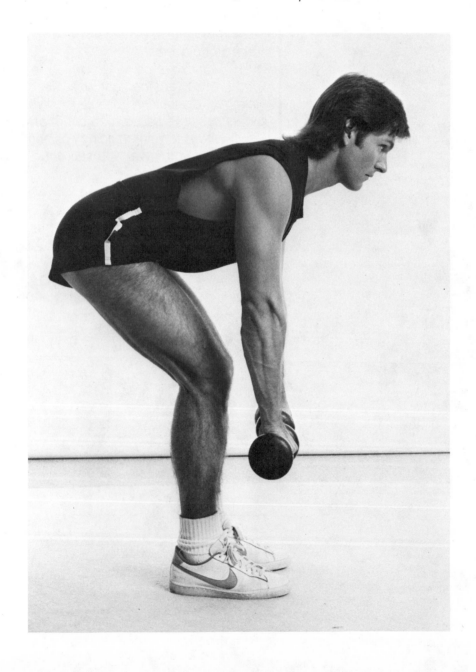

At this point your hands should be in front of you with your arms in a hanging position. Raise your arms by bending your elbows until the upper arms are parallel to the floor. Then slowly lower the dumbbells to the starting position. Do not let the weights touch the floor. Remember to keep your back and neck straight.

Exhale as you pull your arms upward and inhale as you lower your arms.

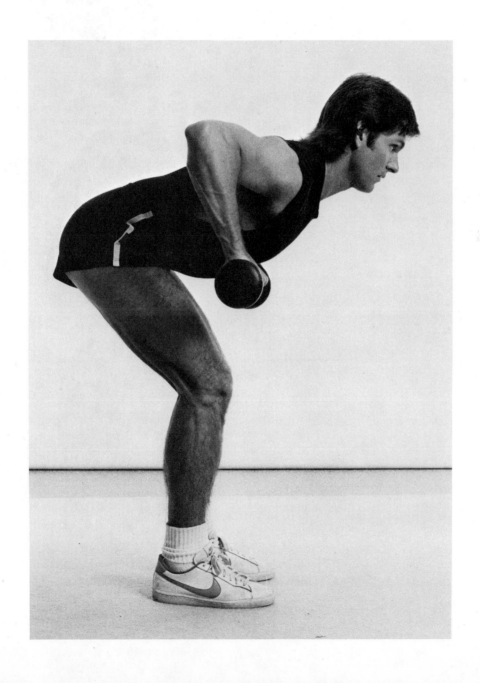

SHRUG ROLL

1 set
15 repetitions

Shrug rolls are a great way to develop and strengthen your upper back muscles. Stand, holding the five- or ten-pound dumbbells at your sides. Position your feet so they are about shoulder-width apart. Stand with your back straight, eyes looking forward, and shoulders slightly back. The dumbbells should be alongside your legs.

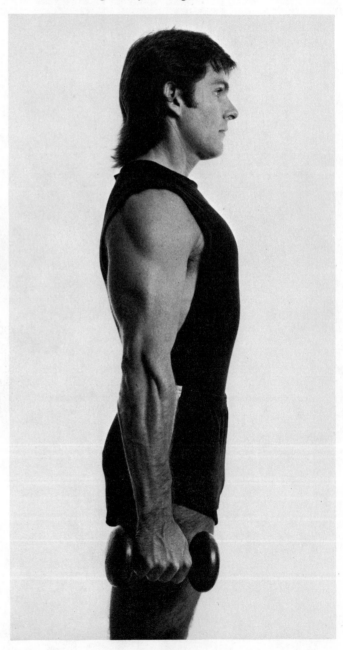

Begin the exercise by raising your shoulders toward your ears. Make sure you do not bend your elbows. When your shoulders are in the "up" position at the top of the shrug, begin to roll your shoulders back and downward by slightly pressing your shoulder blades together. At this point your elbows will bend slightly as your shoulders drop into the starting position.

Exhale when your shoulders are in the up position and inhale as you return to the starting position.

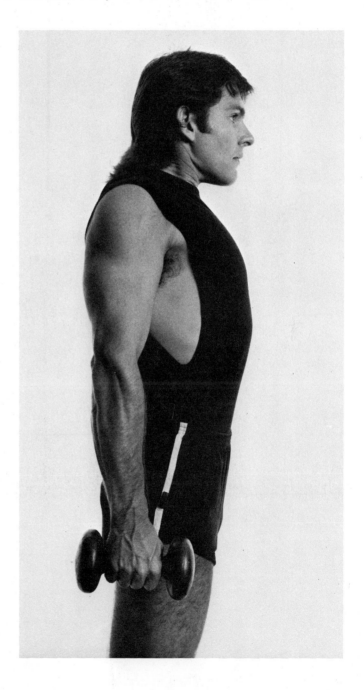

Shoulders and Arms

FRONT LATERAL RAISES

1 set
15 repetitions each arm

The shoulder or deltoid muscle is composed of three different sections. A great exercise for the front part of the shoulder is the front lateral raise.

Stand with the two-and-a-half-pound ankle weights or dumbbells held in your fists with your back and legs in a straight position. With elbows slightly bent, raise your right arm so your hand is level with your shoulder. Return to the starting position and immediately begin the same movement with the left arm. Do fifteen repetitions with each arm, alternating sides. Make sure that you do not swing during this movement.

Exhale as your arms reach the top of the movement, inhale as you lower your arms.

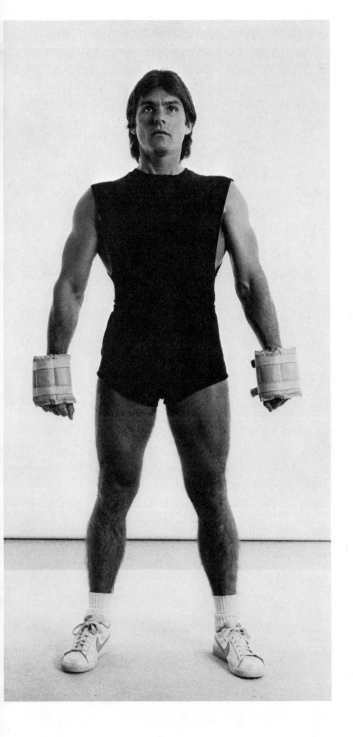

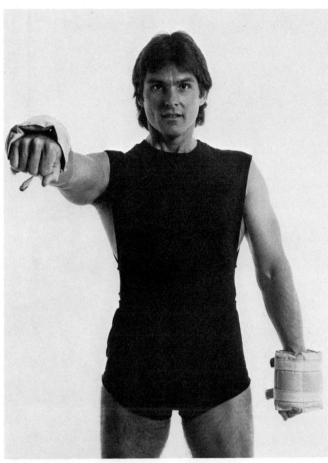

LATERAL RAISES

1 set
15 repetitions

Lateral raises primarily work the side of your shoulder muscle.

To begin, hold the two-and-a-half-pound ankle weights in each fist. Stand with your feet shoulder-width apart. Raise the weights to the top of your shoulders with palms facing the floor. Keep your arms parallel to the floor. Bring your hands down to the side of your thighs, then begin the next repetition.

Exhale as your arms reach the top of the movement, inhale as you lower your arms.

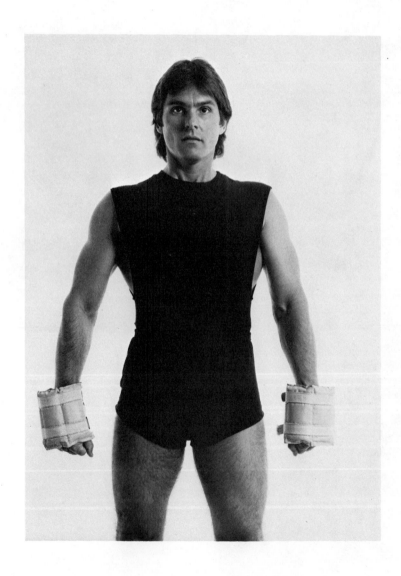

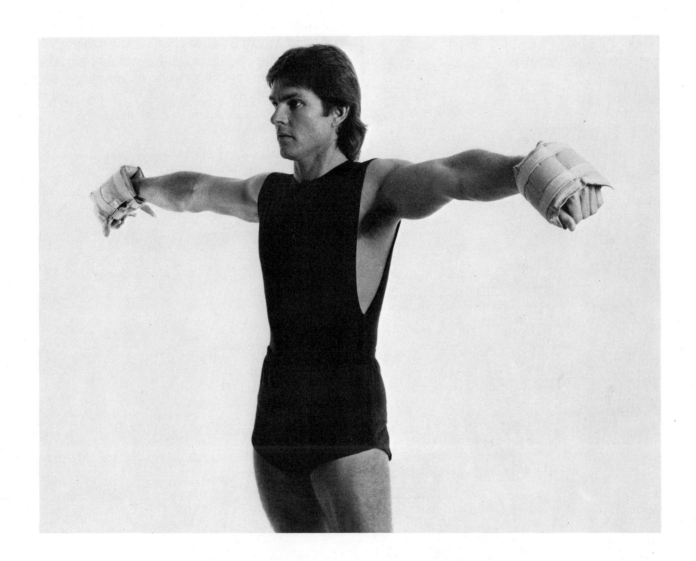

SEATED BENT LATERAL RAISES

1 set
15 repetitions

Bent lateral raises strengthen the rear deltoid muscle or back of your shoulder. Sit on the end of the flat bench, toes and knees together. Bend forward until your lower stomach touches your upper legs. Your head should be raised, your arms hanging, the two two-and-a-half-pound ankle weights close together with the palms of your hands facing each other.

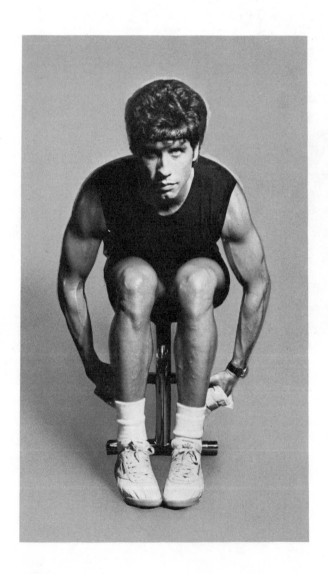

Begin the exercise by slightly bending your elbows. Raise both weights out to the side until they are even with your head. As your arms reach the top of the movement your back and head will raise slightly and your shoulder blades will move together slightly. Lower the weights slowly. Just before the weights touch each other in the down position begin the next repetition.

Exhale as you reach the top of the upward movement. Inhale as you lower the weights.

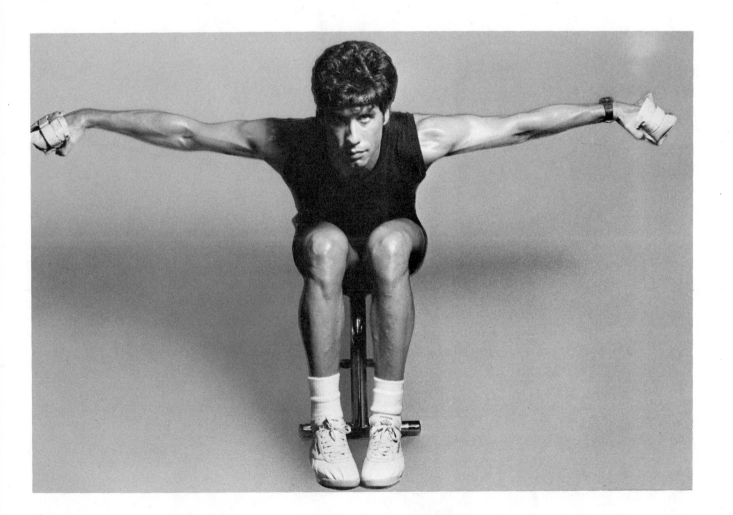

TRICEPS EXTENSION

1 set
15 repetitions

This is a great exercise for developing and toning the entire triceps muscle. The triceps (back of the upper arm) are used in all extension movements. Use the two-and-a-half-pound weights for this exercise.

Lie on the bench in a supine or face-up position with ankle weights in clenched fists, knees bent and

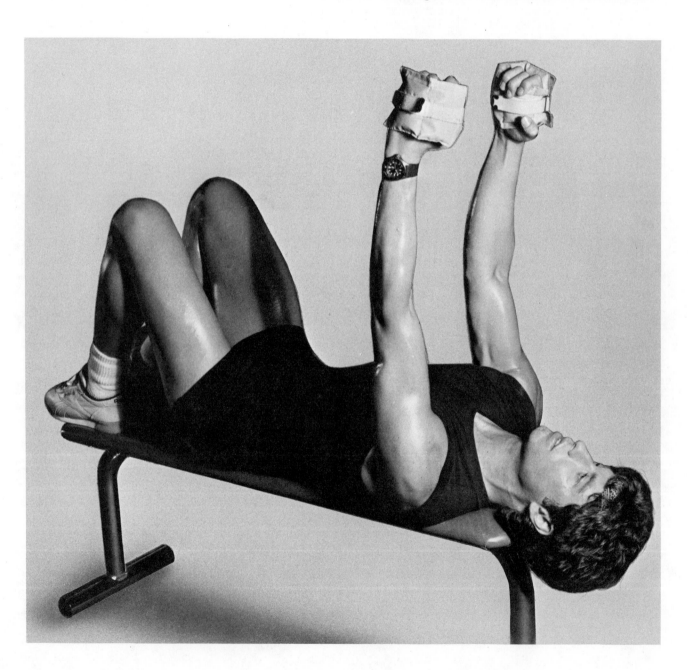

feet flat on the bench. Your head should extend over the edge of the bench. Start with your arms extended straight up toward the ceiling. Keep your upper arms held in place as you lower your hands below your neck. Raise your hands by pressing up to the starting position. Make sure you keep your elbows in a stationary position throughout the exercise.

Exhale as you extend your arms upward, inhale as you lower your arms.

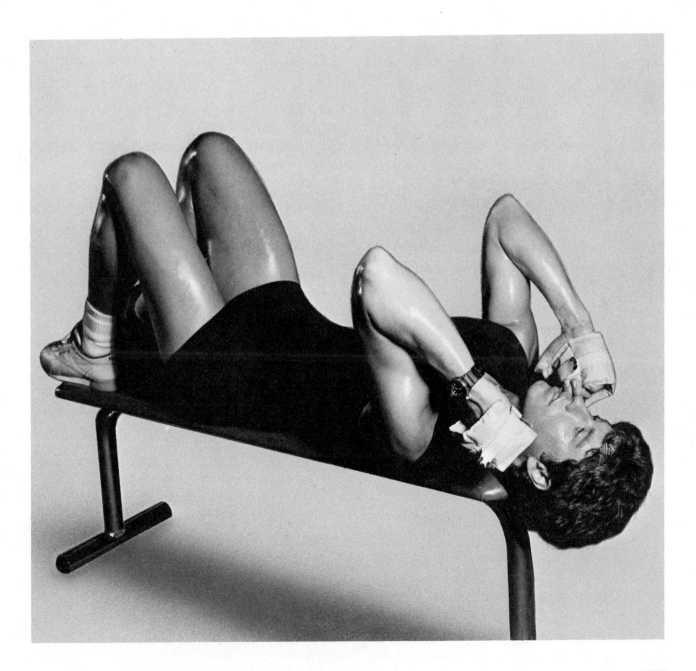

SEATED CURL

1 set
15 repetitions

The seated curl is an excellent way to strengthen the front part of your arms. It will also strengthen your forearms and wrists. Use the five- or ten-pound dumbbells or ankle weights for this exercise.

Sit on the bench with your back straight and feet flat on the floor. Grip the weights firmly with your arms hanging at your sides. Turn your palms so they are facing forward, bend your elbows, and curl your forearms to your shoulders. Squeeze your biceps at the top of the movement. This will fully contract the biceps muscle. Then lower your arms, turning your palms in toward your legs to starting position. Be sure to keep your back straight and shoulders stationary during this exercise. Do fifteen repetitions with both arms simultaneously.

Exhale as you curl your arms upward and inhale as your arms return to the starting position.

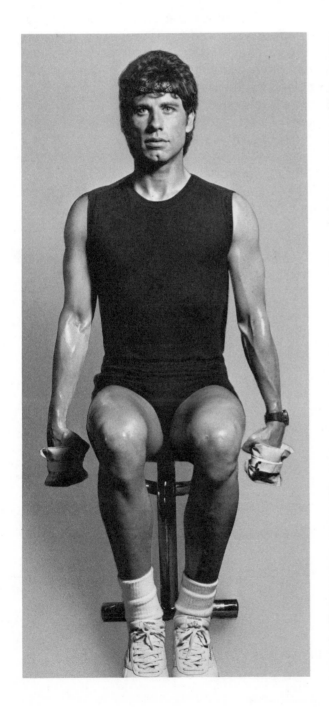
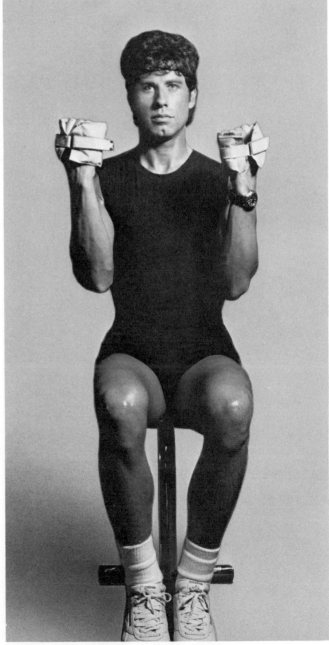

Intermediate Program

45 MINUTES
45 SECONDS BETWEEN SETS
3 DAYS PER WEEK

Abdominals

BENT LEG SIT-UPS

2 sets
30 repetitions

Set sit-up board at a slight angle—your head will be at the lower end. Sit on the board with your knees bent, your insteps pressed against the pad, and your knees and toes pressed together. Fold your hands against your chest. I begin my sit-ups in the "up" position with my stomach flexed because it places less initial strain on my lower back.

Begin the exercise by lowering your body until your lower back touches the board. Return only one third of the distance to an upright position, about a 30-degree arc, for each repetition. Use a moderate speed for this exercise.

Exhale as you begin to sit up and inhale as you return to the starting position.

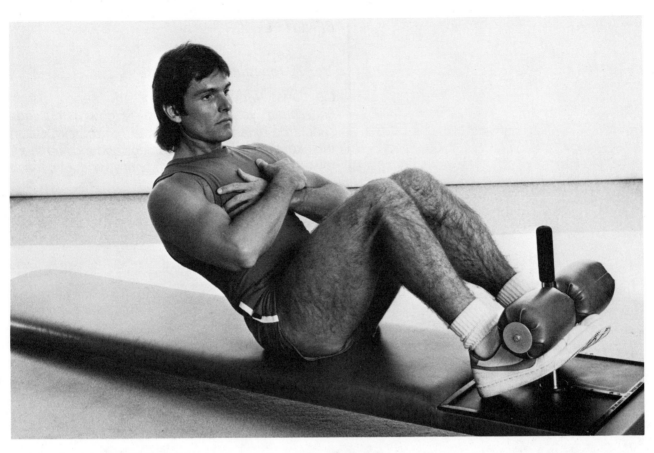

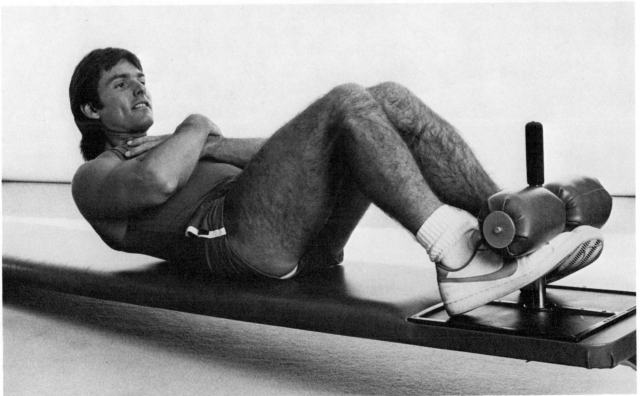

BENCH FLEXOR

2 sets
30 repetitions

Lie down with your back on the bench, hands underneath your buttocks, palms down. Your legs should be extended straight out horizontally. Begin the exercise by bending your legs and moving them toward your chest. Continue until your thighs touch

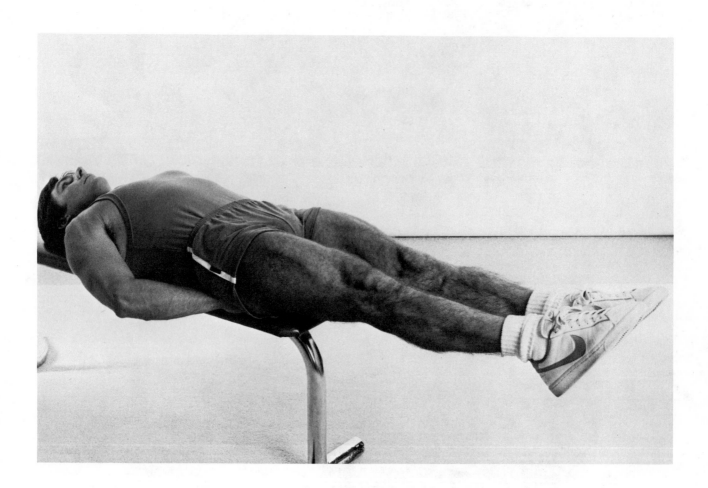

the lower part of your stomach, then return to the starting position. Point your toes when you extend your legs, flex your feet when you bend your legs.

Exhale as your legs move toward your chest. Inhale as you return to the starting position.

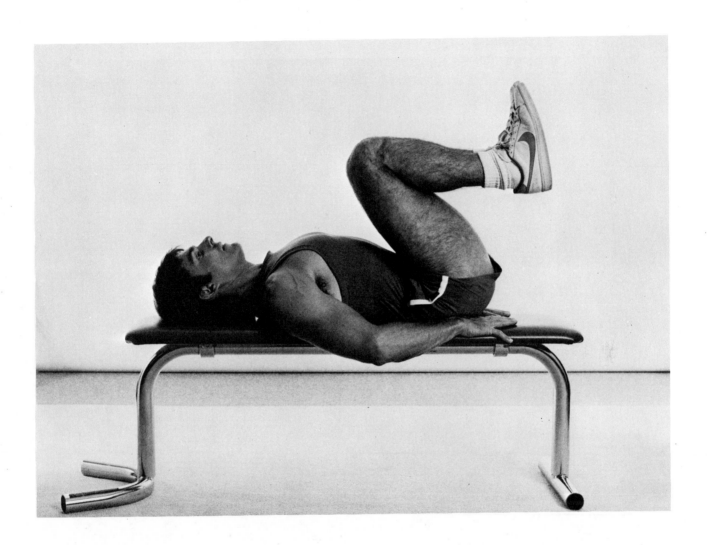

ALTERNATE LEG LIFTS

2 sets
50 repetitions

Lie on the floor with your hands underneath your buttocks, palms down. Raise your legs six inches off the floor. Your feet should be pointed.

Begin by raising your right leg approximately a foot and a half above the left leg, then return it to

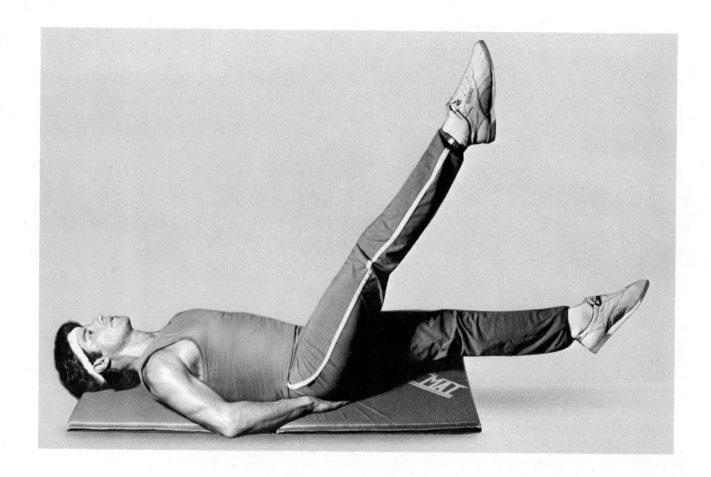

the starting position while simultaneously raising the left leg. Each leg movement is counted as one repetition. Use a fast speed for this exercise.

Inhale and exhale for every two repetitions. Try to breathe as naturally and rhythmically as possible during the exercise.

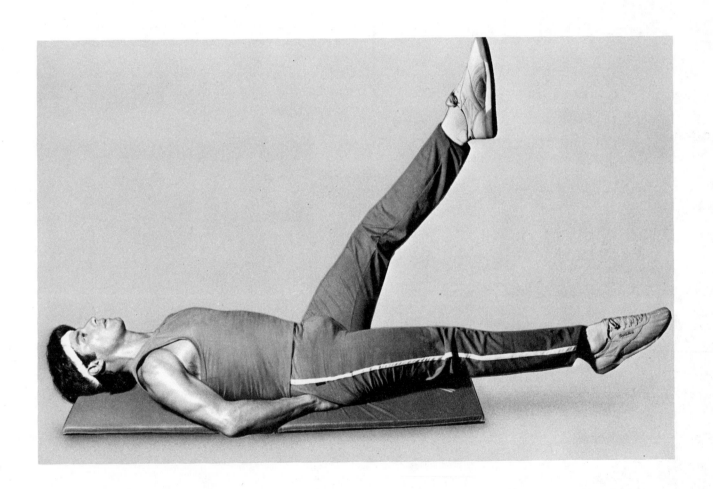

Chest

PULL-OVERS

> *2 sets*
> *12 repetitions*

Use a five- or ten-pound dumbbell for this exercise. Grip the dumbbell at one end with both hands. Lie down with your back on the bench, your head extended over the edge and your feet flat on the bench. Straighten your arms by pushing your hands toward the ceiling. Slowly lower your arms behind your head until they are below your head—your arms will bend slightly. Bring your arms back into starting position by pulling with your chest muscles. This exercise will expand your rib cage and chest area.

Inhale as you lower the dumbbell, exhale as you raise it.

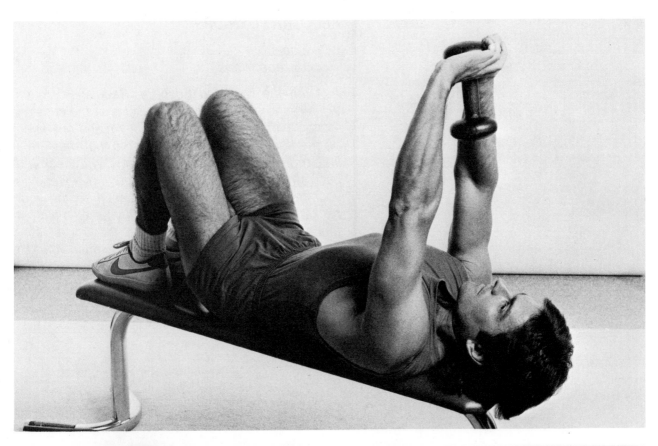

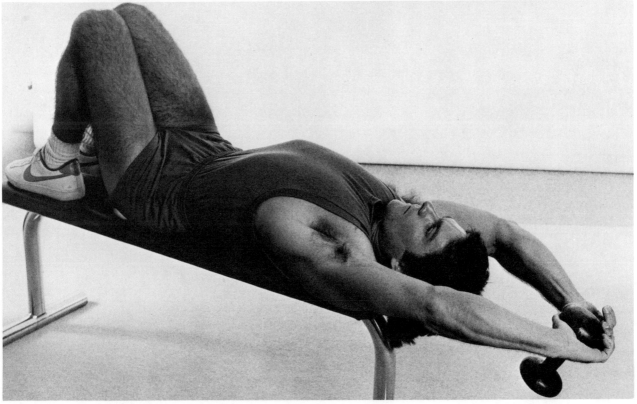

REGULAR PUSH-UPS

2 sets
15 repetitions

As with the Modified Push-up, Regular Push-ups will strengthen the pectoral muscles of the chest.

Start with your hands palms down and one knee on the floor. Position your hands so that they are a little more than shoulder-width apart, with neck and back straight. Begin in the up position by extending your resting leg into a straight line. Keeping your back straight, lower yourself until your chin almost touches the floor, then return to the up position, squeezing your chest together as you push yourself upward.

Inhale as you move toward the floor. Exhale as you push away from the floor.

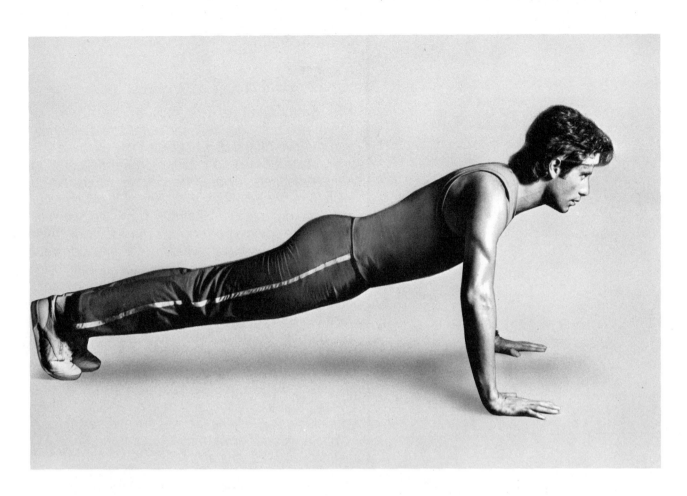

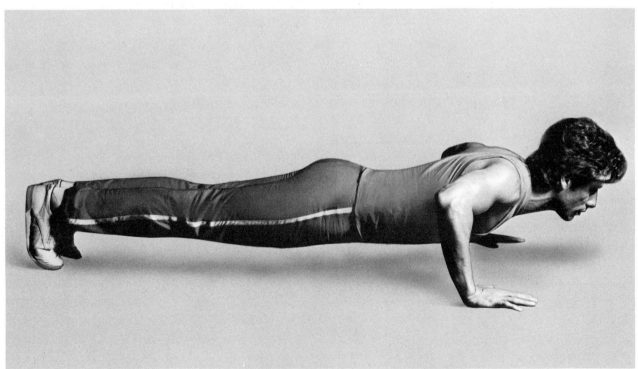

CROSS-OVERS

2 sets
12 repetitions

The Cross-Over exercise is a great way to strengthen both the inner and outer chest muscles. Use the five-pound dumbbells for this exercise. Lie in a supine or face-up position on the bench, with arms extended toward the ceiling, palms facing each other. Begin the exercise by bending your arms and dropping your elbows below the bench as if you were doing a butterfly movement. The dumbbells should be parallel to the floor as you drop your elbows. Return your arms toward the starting position, moving the dumbbells back in a hugging, semicircular manner. Just before you reach the starting position, turn your hands so the palms face out and the dumbbells are allowed to cross. Cross your forearms as you squeeze your chest muscles together, then move the dumbbells back to the starting position again, turning your palms so they face one another as you begin the next repetition. Keep your elbows slightly bent throughout the exercise.

Inhale as your arms move toward the floor. Exhale as you raise your arms.

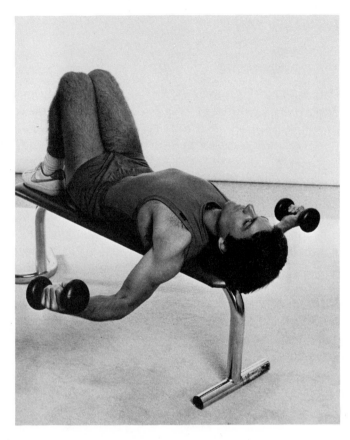

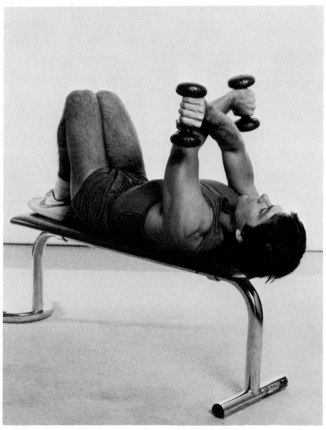

PARALLEL BAR DIPS

2 sets
12 repetitions

Parallel-bar Dips are great for chest development. They particularly work the lower and outer chest muscles. Your hands should be facing each other as you face into the dip station.

Begin the exercise in an up position with arms slightly bent and chest forward, legs bent behind you. Remember to keep your head and chest forward throughout the movement. Bend your elbows pushing your chest forward and legs slightly backward, until your arms form at least a 90-degree angle. Try to slowly stretch this movement past the 90-degree angle if possible before returning to the starting position. Squeeze your chest muscles together at the top of the movement.

Inhale as you move downward and exhale as you push yourself upward.

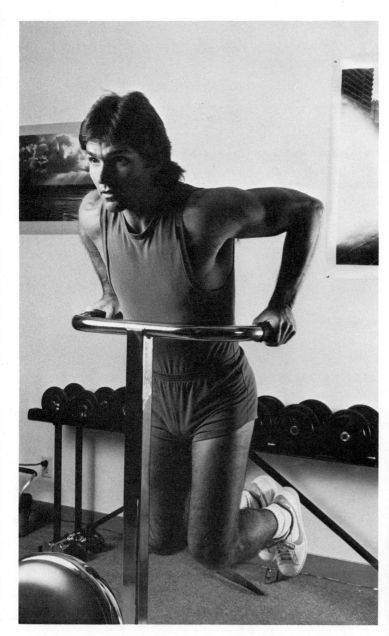

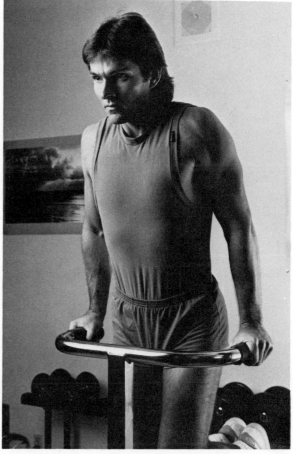

Back

SHRUG

2 sets
12 repetitions

This is a movement similar to the Shrug Roll used in the beginners program for upper back development. Use five- or ten-pound dumbbells for this exercise.

Stand with your feet shoulder-width apart, arms at your sides, back straight and eyes forward. The dumbbells should be slightly behind your legs.

From this starting position begin to raise your shoulders toward your ears. Make sure you do not bend your elbows during the movement. Pause for a count of one at the top before lowering your shoulders to the starting position.

Exhale toward the top of the shrug movement, and inhale as your shoulders are lowered to the starting position.

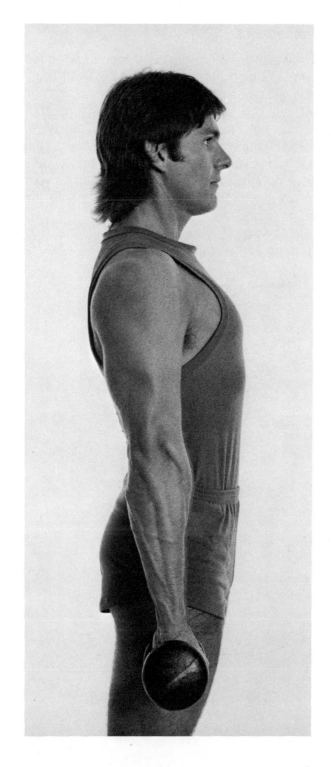
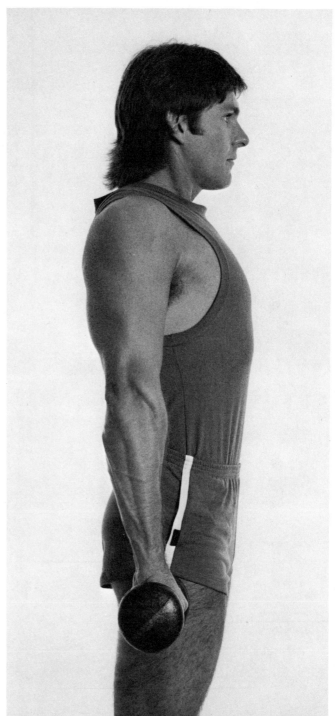

PULL-UPS

2 sets
5 repetitions

Pull-ups are a great way to give your back added width and develop the latissimus dorsi or lat muscles. You will use a chin-up bar for this exercise.

Grip the bar with your palms facing forward. Your grip should be a little wider than shoulder-width apart. Raise yourself by pulling your body up to the bar, then cross your chin over the bar. Your elbows will move downward and slightly backward as your legs move slightly backward. Slowly return to the starting position.

Exhale as you pull yourself up and inhale as you are returning to the starting position.

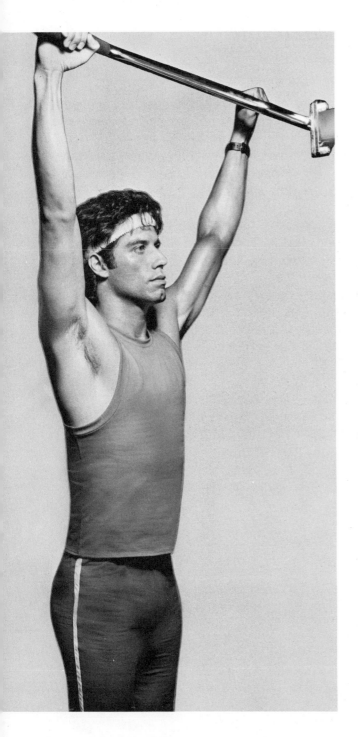

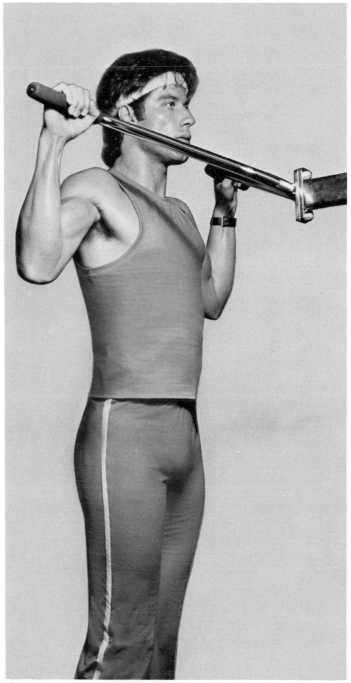

DUMBBELL DEAD LIFT

2 sets
12 repetitions

For the intermediate program we will again use the Dead-Lift exercise. It is a hard exercise to bypass for lower back work. Use the five- or ten-pound dumbbells for this exercise. Remember what I said earlier about slightly bending your knees, even though I often keep mine straight!

Stand with your feet shoulder-width apart, your legs slightly bent, and dumbbells at your sides.

To begin the exercise, bend your upper body over as though you were touching your toes. During the movement the dumbbell heads should be about four inches apart. As you reach the lowest point, roll your shoulders back to help maintain your back in a straight line. When you reach your full stretch, begin to raise your upper body back to the starting position.

Do this exercise slowly, making sure to use your lower back muscles.

Inhale as you bend over and exhale as you pull the weight upward to the starting position.

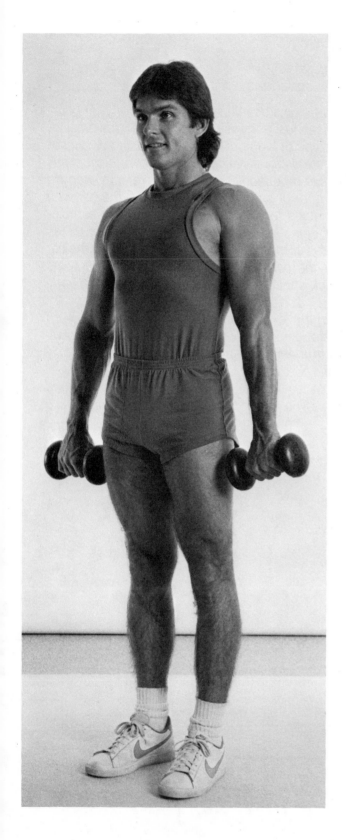

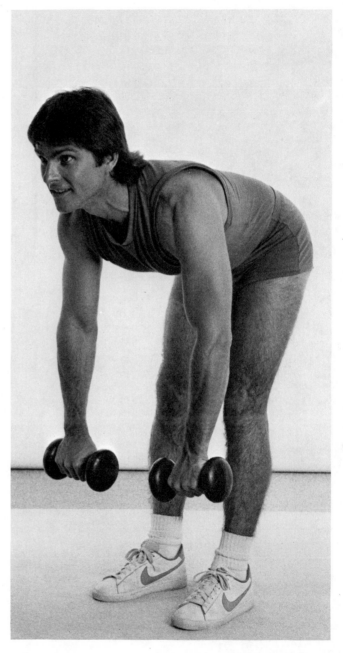

PULL-DOWNS

2 sets
12 repetitions

Lat Pull-Downs develop the large part of your back, the latissimus dorsi muscles. Use a Universal or similar type of high pulley. Begin by using twenty or thirty pounds, or a weight you can comfortably pull for twelve repetitions. You do this exercise kneeling on the floor or sitting on a bench. Grip the bar with palms facing forward. Your grip should be approximately eight inches beyond each shoulder or as wide as is comfortably possible. Kneel under the bar so that the bar is directly behind your head. Arms and back should be aligned, and your head slightly forward.

Begin by evenly pulling the weight downward until it touches the back of your neck. Then slowly return to the starting position letting your arms fully extend.

Exhale as you pull the weight downward and inhale as you return to the starting position.

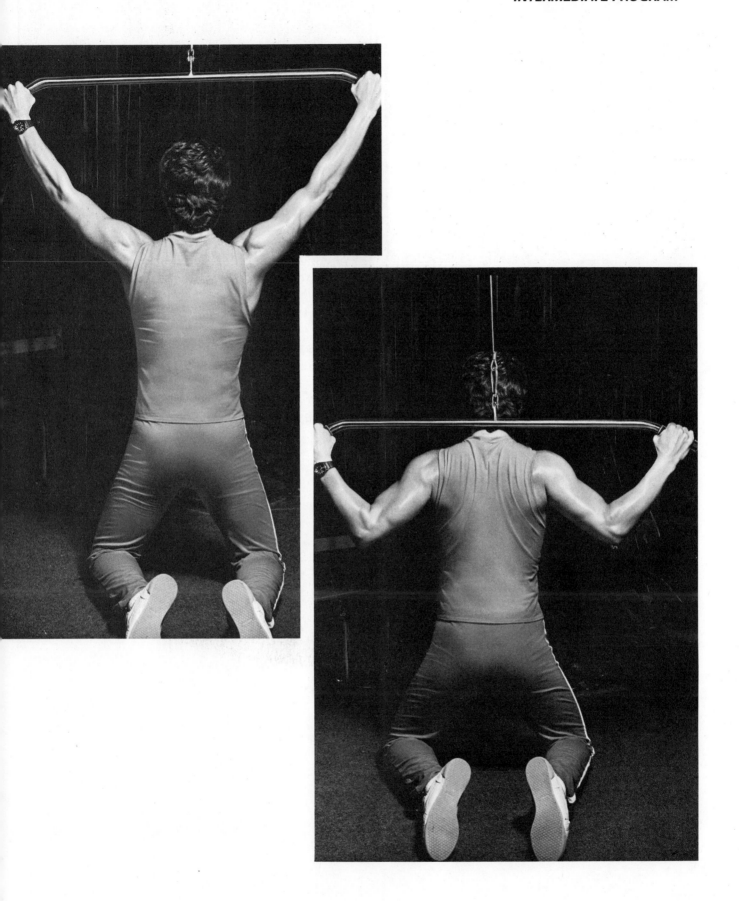

Shoulders and Arms

FRONT SHOULDER PRESS

2 sets
12 repetitions

The Front Shoulder Press is a great way to strengthen the front deltoid muscle. Use the shoulder press for this exercise. Start with twenty or thirty pounds or a weight you can comfortably press for twelve repetitions.

Begin by sitting on a bench facing the machine. Your shoulders should be level with the handles of the machine, your back and head in a straight position. Firmly grip the middle of each handle.

Push the weight upward and slightly forward until your arms are fully extended, then lower your arms by dropping your elbows. Continue as far as possible or until the weight touches the stack, then begin the next repetition.

Exhale as you press the weight upward, inhale as you lower the weight.

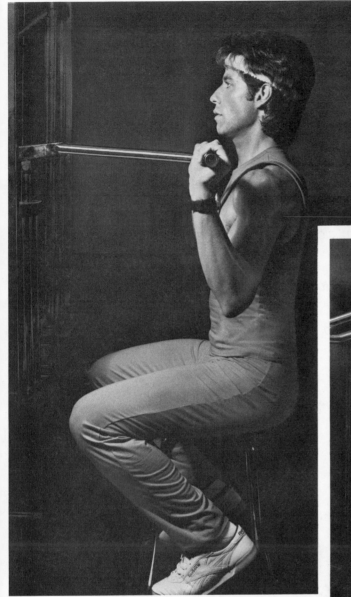

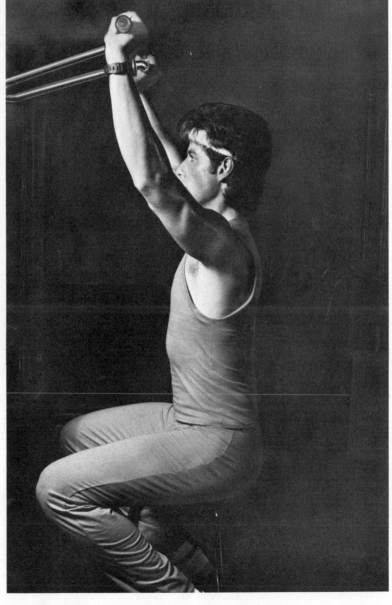

LATERAL RAISES

2 sets
12 repetitions

Lateral Raises develop the side shoulder muscle. Use the five-pound dumbbells.

Begin by standing with your legs slightly bent. With a five-pound dumbbell in each hand stand with feet shoulder-width apart, hands at your sides, palms facing your legs. Raise the weights to the side until they are even with the top of your shoulders, slightly pushing your wrists toward the ceiling. Keep the dumbbells parallel to the floor at all times. Then slowly lower your arms to the starting position.

Exhale as you raise your arms upward and inhale as you lower your arms.

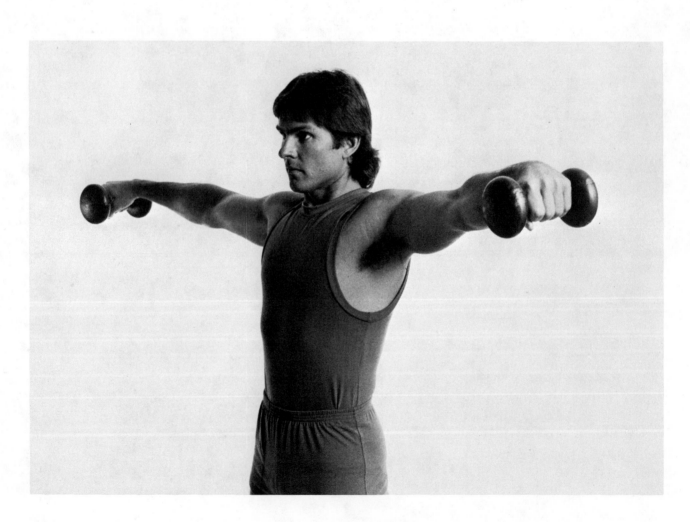

STANDING BENT LATERAL RAISES

2 sets
12 repetitions

Bent Lateral Raises develop the rear deltoid muscle of the shoulder. Use five- or ten-pound dumbbells.

Place your feet approximately shoulder-width apart. Your arms should be hanging at your sides. Grip the dumbbells so that your palms are facing each other. Slightly bend your knees for this exercise. Bend your torso until it is parallel to the floor. Arms should be in front of your body, the dumbbells in front of your legs approximately four inches apart.

Keeping your back straight, raise your arms sideways until the dumbbells are even with your head. Then slowly lower them to the starting position. Keep a slight bend in your elbows while raising the dumbbells.

Exhale as you raise your arms and inhale as you lower your arms.

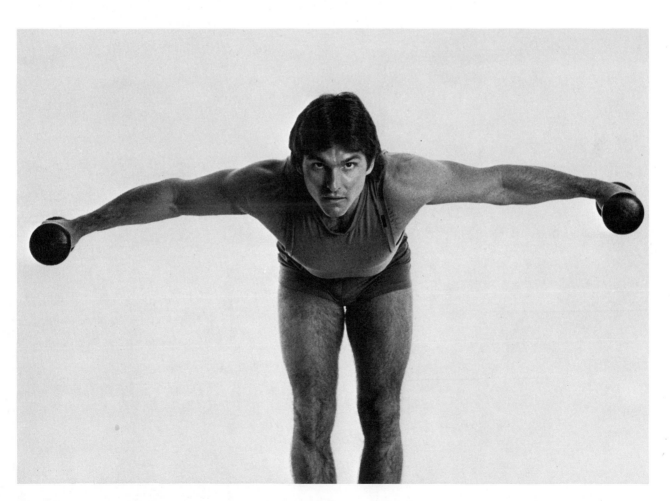

DIPS (TRICEPS)

2 sets
12 repetitions

Dips are a perfect exercise for the entire triceps muscle. For this exercise you will be using the bench.

Grip the side of the bench with both hands and extend your legs in front, with your heels against the floor and your buttocks raised slightly off the bench. Keep your arms and back straight. Lower your buttocks toward the floor by bending your elbows as much as possible. Then raise your buttocks to the starting position by pressing down on the bench, using the back of your arms. Press until your arms are again extended.

Keep your back and neck straight throughout the movement. Make sure the bench cannot slip.

Inhale as you lower yourself and exhale as you push yourself upward.

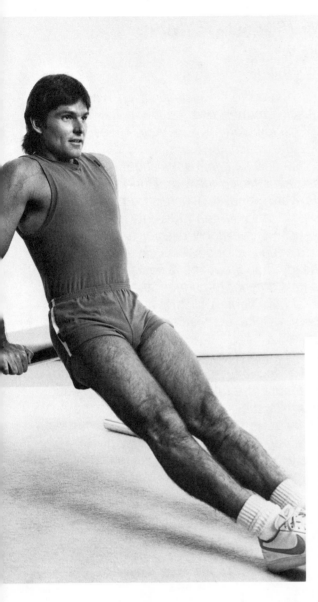

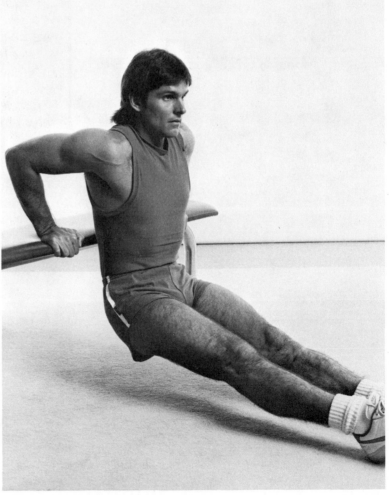

KNEELING TRICEPS EXTENSION

2 sets
12 repetitions

This exercise is a great variation which works the triceps muscle. You will use the low pulley for this exercise. Position yourself on your knees facing away from the machine. I am using a Universal machine. Use a close grip, hands about four inches apart, with palms facing forward. Elbows should be pointing forward, about two inches from either side of your head. Start with ten to twenty pounds, or a weight you can comfortably use for twelve repetitions. Try to keep your elbows as close as possible to your head throughout the exercise. Your back should be held straight throughout the exercise and your head should be in a slightly forward position. Your elbows will be bent at approximately a 90-degree angle.

Keeping your upper arms stationary, straighten your elbows and extend your forearms straight overhead. Just before fully locking your elbows out, slowly return to the starting position. Let the bar extend as far as is comfortable, usually about ear level, before beginning the next extension.

Exhale as you extend your arms and inhale as you return to the starting position.

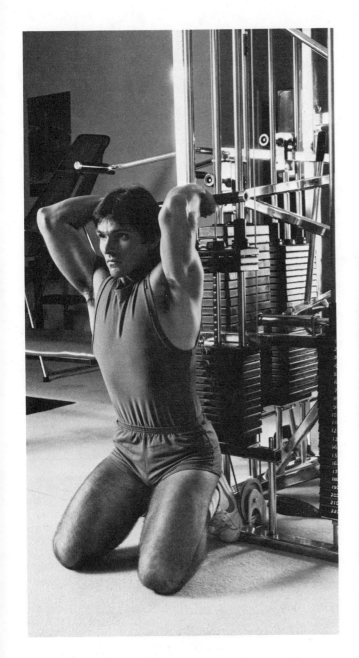

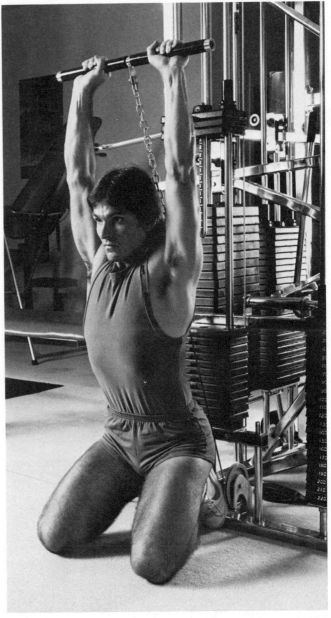

HAMMERHEAD ALTERNATE CURLS

2 sets
12 repetitions, each arm, alternating

The Hammerhead Alternate Curl works the entire biceps muscle as well as the forearm.

Grip a five- or ten-pound dumbbell in each hand, with palms facing in toward the body. Your back should be straight, your eyes looking forward. Keep your elbows as close to your sides as possible.

Begin with your right arm and curl the weight toward your shoulder, squeezing your biceps at the top of the movement, then slowly return to the starting position. Alternate arms for twelve repetitions each.

Exhale as you curl each arm upward and inhale as you lower each arm.

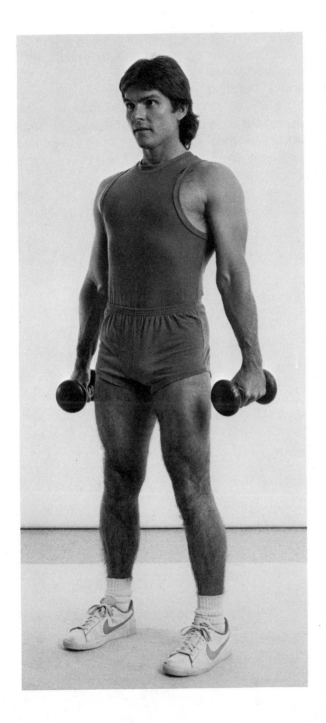
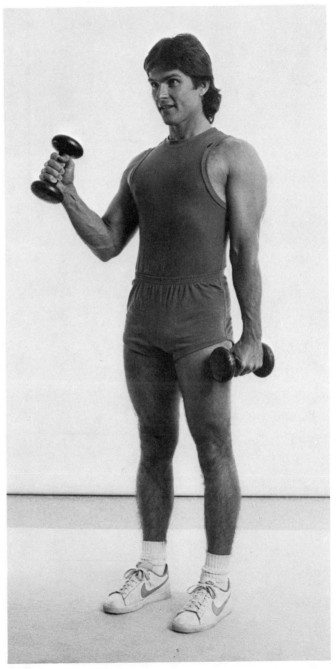

PULLEY CURL

2 sets
12 repetitions

The Pulley Curl is a great exercise for the biceps muscle. I am using a Universal machine. You will be using the low pulley for this exercise. Begin with ten to twenty pounds, or a weight you can comfortably pull for twelve repetitions.

Facing the machine, hold the bar with a close grip, palms up and hands about four inches apart. Position yourself so your arms are fully extended, with your back held straight and shoulders back.

Begin by bending your forearms upward. Curl both arms up, moving your hands as close as possible toward your shoulders, and squeeze your biceps at the top of the movement. Then slowly lower your arms until they are full extended. Keep your elbows in at your sides.

Exhale as you curl your hands upward and inhale as you lower your hands to the starting position.

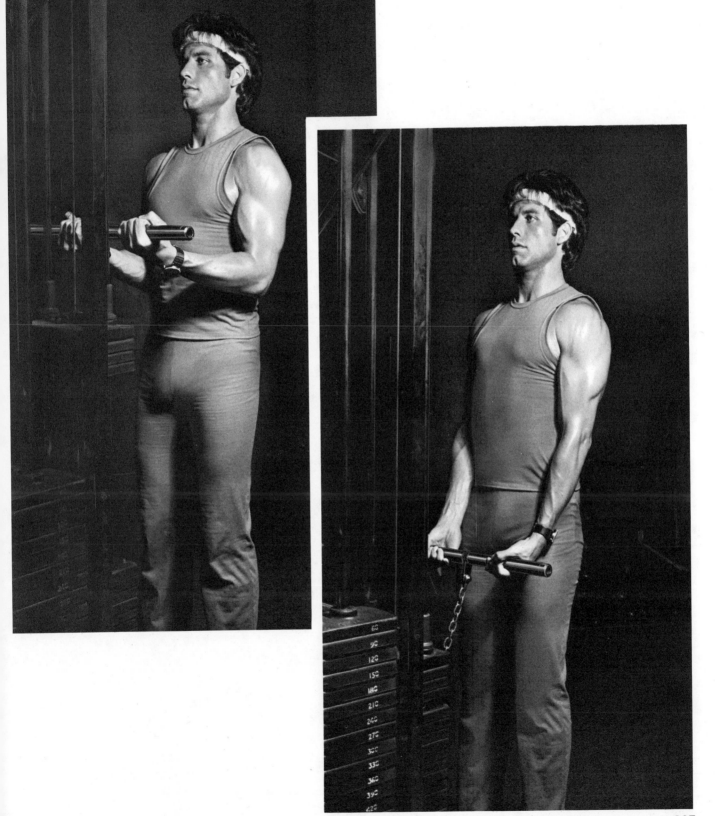

Advanced Program

60 MINUTES
30-45 SECONDS BETWEEN SETS
3 DAYS PER WEEK

ADVANCED WEIGHT TRAINING WARM-UP

After the daily warm-ups (see page 15), those training in the advance program should do an additional warm-up set for the chest, the back, and the shoulders and arms, before beginning the regular workout.

These warm-up sets should be done with a light weight—lighter than the weight you would normally use for each exercise. Choose a weight you can comfortably handle for fifteen repetitions at a moderately fast speed.

These are the warm-ups I recommend:
Chest
*   Bench Press (page 210)—1 set*
Back
*   Pull-Downs (page 220—1 set*
Shoulders and Arms
*   Shoulder Press (page 234)—1 set*
*   Press-Downs (Triceps) (page 236)—1 set*
*   Hammerhead Alternate Curl (Biceps) (page 202)—1 set*

Abdominals

BENT-LEG SIT-UPS

> *3 sets*
> *30 repetitions*

By using an incline board for this exercise, you will be able to isolate and work the abdominal muscles better. Most sit-up boards can be adjusted to several different degrees of incline. Make sure you choose the lowest position first when learning this exercise.

Position yourself on the board so your head is lower than your feet and your insteps are pressed against the strap or cushions. Toes and knees should be pressed together. If you wish you can roll up a towel and place it between your knees. As you perform the exercise you will be squeezing your knees together. This helps to isolate the abdominal muscles.

Begin sitting up with your arms crossed over your chest. In order to increase the effectiveness of the exercise, you can hold a ten-pound weight, as I am in the picture. Eyes should be looking forward with back and neck straight. Lower your upper body until your lower back touches the board. Return only one third of the way toward a full sitting position so that you travel through a 30-degree arc.

Do the exercise with moderate speed, exhaling as you begin to sit forward. Inhale as you lower yourself on the board.

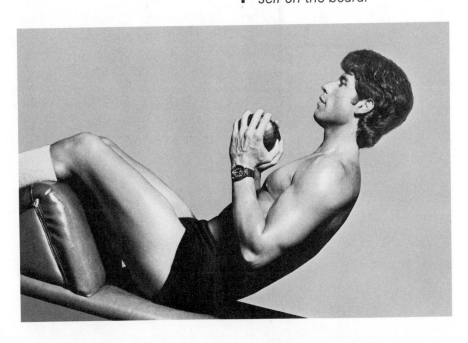

FLEXORS

3 sets
30 repetitions

Flexors will strengthen your lower abdominals. The easiest way to do this exercise is to reverse your position on the sit-up board following your Bent-Leg Sit-ups. Lie on your back with your head at the raised end of the board, chin on your chest. Your legs should be together with feet flexed and your hands should grip the top handle of the board.

Raise your legs so that your feet are approximately six inches off the board. Begin the exercise by bending your knees and moving them toward your chest. Continue until the small of your back is off the board, then return to the starting position with feet six inches off the board. Keep your feet flexed throughout the exercise.

Exhale as your legs move toward your chest and inhale as you move back to the starting position.

BICYCLES

1 set
100 repetitions

Lie on a mat with hands clasped behind your head, back straight, legs and head raised off the floor. Begin by touching your right elbow to your left knee, simultaneously fully extending your right leg. Make sure your legs remain off the floor throughout the exercise. Then touch your left elbow to your right knee, and straighten your left leg. Keep your upper back slightly off the floor. Do fifty repetitions with feet flexed and fifty repetitions with feet pointed. You can work up to using the two-and-a-half-pound ankle weights for this exercise.

Use a moderately fast speed with this exercise. One repetition consists of touching one elbow to the opposite knee. Exhale when each knee is in the back position. Inhale in between movements.

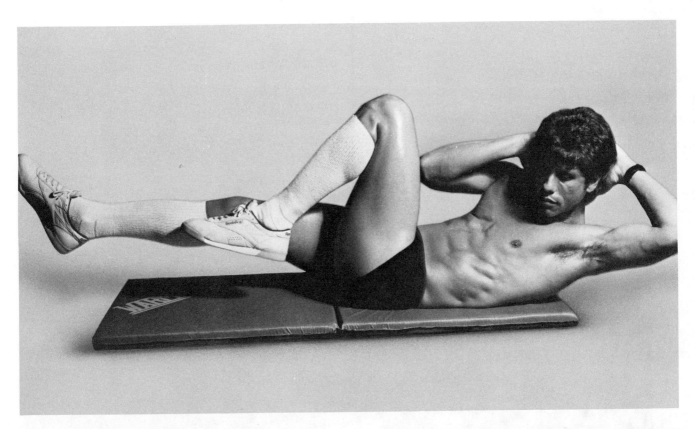

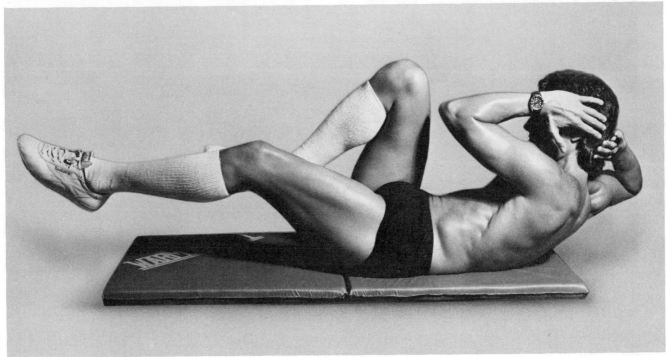

Chest

BENCH PRESS

> *3 sets*
> *10 repetitions*

This is the best exercise for developing the overall chest or pectoral muscles. When working without a partner it is best to use a Universal, Paramount, or a similar type of machine.

Lie down on the bench in a supine or face-up position. The bar handles should be even with your nipples. Feet should be flat on the floor. Grip the handles in the middle with a firm grip. Begin with a

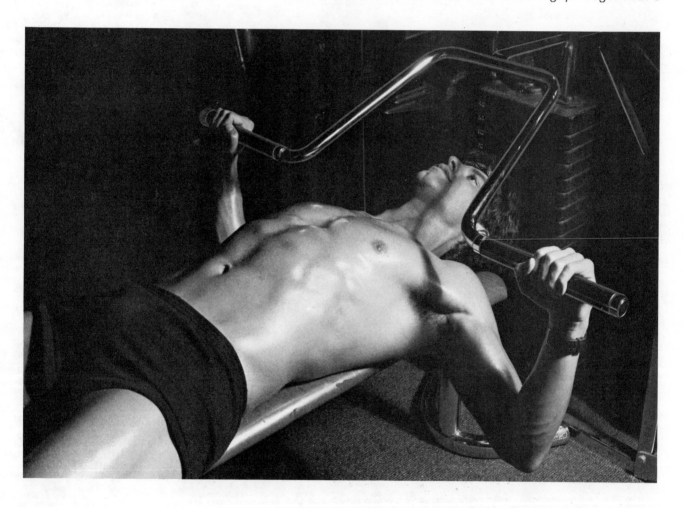

weight that you can comfortably press for ten repetitions.

Begin the exercise by pushing the weight upward. Slowly lower the weight to the starting position by dropping your elbows below your back, pushing your chest upward as you lower the weight. As the weight touches the stack immediately begin your next repetition. If your back begins to arch, put your feet flat on the bench.

Exhale as you push the weight upward and inhale as you lower the weight.

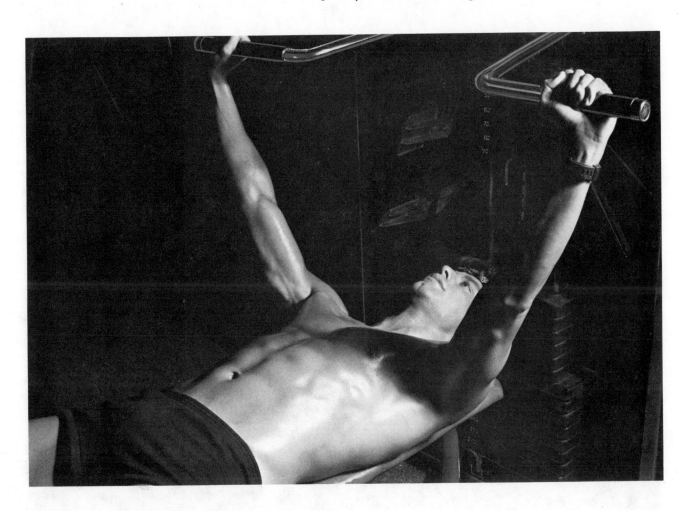

INCLINE BENCH PRESS

3 sets
10 repetitions

As we raise the head of the bench we will work the upper pectoral or chest muscle. You may need to use a block of wood to tilt the bench if you do not have an incline bench. Select a weight that you can comfortably press for ten repetitions—a lighter weight than you used for the Bench Press exercise. Place the head of the bench on top of the block and move the bench so it is about six inches from the machine. Lie on the bench face up, so that the handles are approximately even with your neck. Place your feet on the floor. Again, if your back tends to arch off the bench, bend your knees and

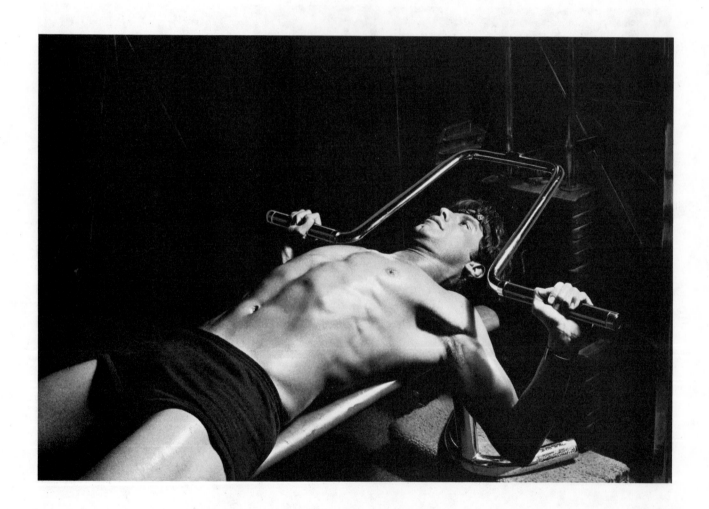

place your feet flat on the bench. Use a mid-sized grip—hands not too wide apart—and grip the bar firmly.

Begin by pressing the weight upward until your arms are fully straightened. Return to the starting position by bending your elbows and slowly lowering the weight. Drop your elbows below your back as far as possible to stretch your pectoral muscles fully, and then begin the next repetition. Push your chest out as you lower the weight.

Exhale as you push the weight up and inhale as you let the weight down.

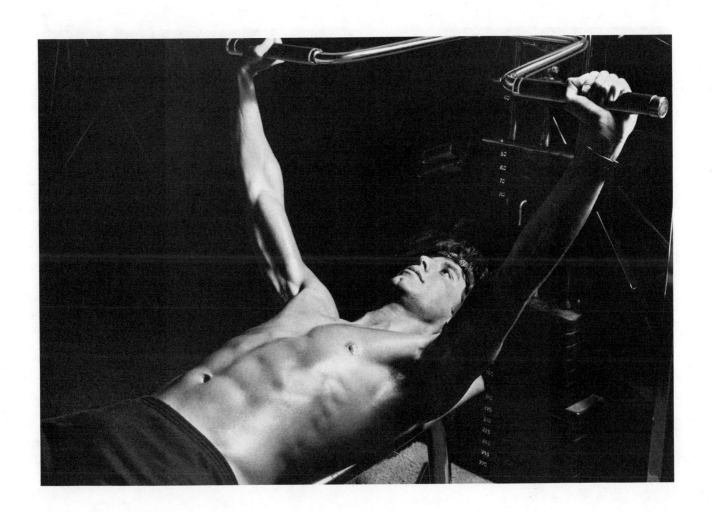

DECLINE BENCH PRESS

3 sets
10 repetitions

Now that you have trained the mid- and upper sections of your chest, you need to work the lower area. Use the same block of wood you used for the Incline Bench Press. This time, however, place the block under the foot of the bench. The head of the bench should be against the machine. Select a weight that you can comfortably press for ten repetitions.

Lie on the bench face up. The handles should be about two inches below your nipples. Again, if you feel your back arching, place your feet flat on the

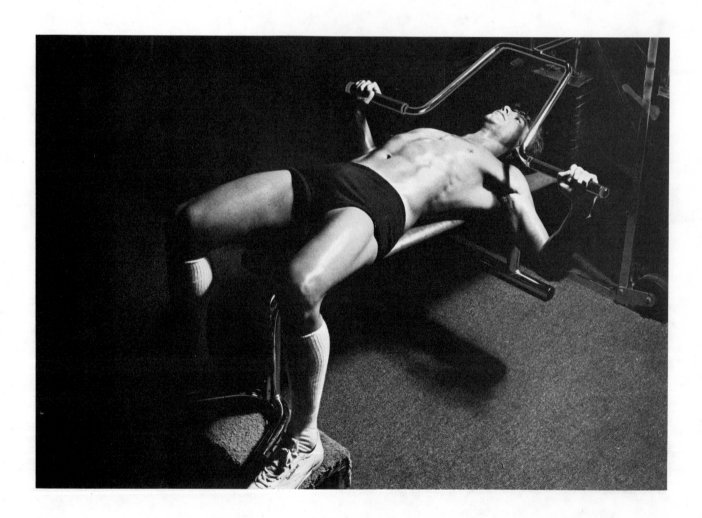

bench rather than on the floor. Grip each handle firmly.

Begin by pressing the weight upward. Extend until your arms are straightened, then slowly lower the weight by dropping your elbows below your back. Push your chest out as you lower the weight. Stretch your chest as far as possible before beginning the next repetition.

Exhale as you push the weight up and inhale as you lower it.

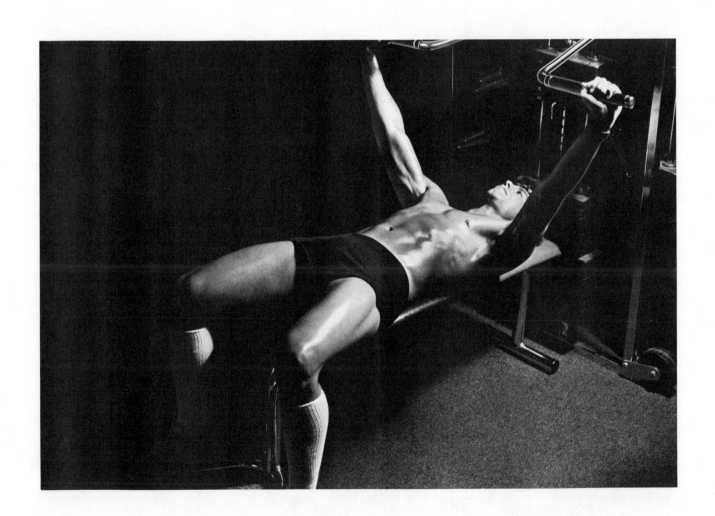

DUMBBELL FLYS

3 sets
10 repetitions

Flys are a great way to work the outside of your pectoral muscles. Use a flat bench for this exercise. Begin with five- or ten-pound dumbbells, working up to heavier weights gradually.

Lie on the bench in a face-up or supine position. Your arms are to the sides, extended upward and slightly bent, with palms facing each other. Feet should be on the floor.

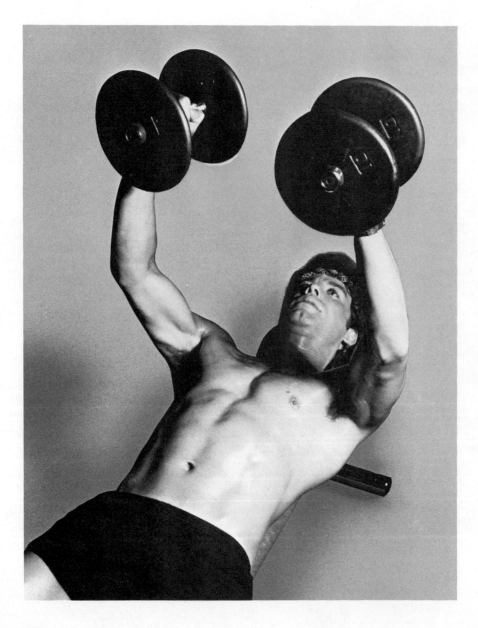

Begin the exercise by lowering the dumbbells until your elbows are slightly below your back. Your chest will be pushed upward during this movement. As you begin to raise your arms, concentrate on your chest muscles. Press your arms upward with a hugging movement. At the top of the movement, flex your chest muscles together but do not let the dumbbell heads touch, then immediately begin the next repetition. Make sure you keep the dumbbells parallel to the floor at all times.

Exhale as you push the weights upward and together. Inhale as you lower them.

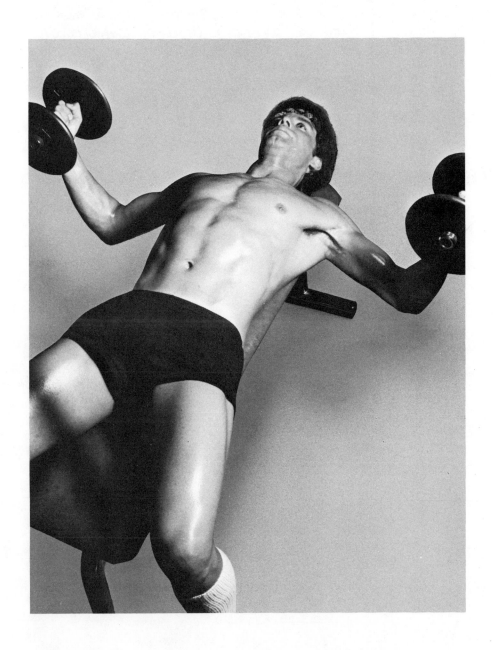

PULL-OVERS

3 sets
10 repetitions

Pull-Overs are the perfect way to complete your chest workout. They will expand the rib cage as well as tone and stretch the abdominal muscles. Use a five-pound weight to start.

Lie on the bench face up. Grip the dumbbells so that your palms are against the inside of one end of the dumbbell. Raise the dumbbell toward the ceiling with arms straightened.

Begin by lowering your arms past your head, until the top of the dumbbell is even with the back of your head. As you lower your arms, you will have to bend your elbows. Pull the dumbbell back into the starting position, straightening your arms as the weight moves past your face. Your arms will describe a semi-circular motion. Concentrate on letting your chest do the pulling.

Inhale as you lower the weight. Exhale as you raise the weight.

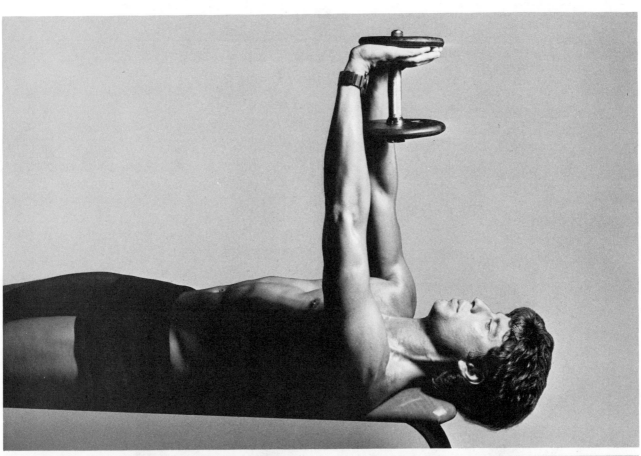

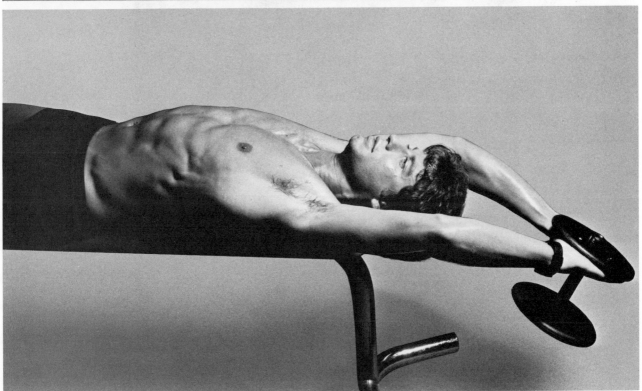

Back

PULL-DOWNS (BACK)

3 sets
10 repetitions

Pull-Downs work your lats or the large section of your back. This first exercise will be completed by pulling the weight down behind your head. (In the next exercise the bar will be pulled down in front of your face.) This will work the upper lats and add width to your back. This is also a great way to start your back workout because it helps to warm up and stretch the entire back.

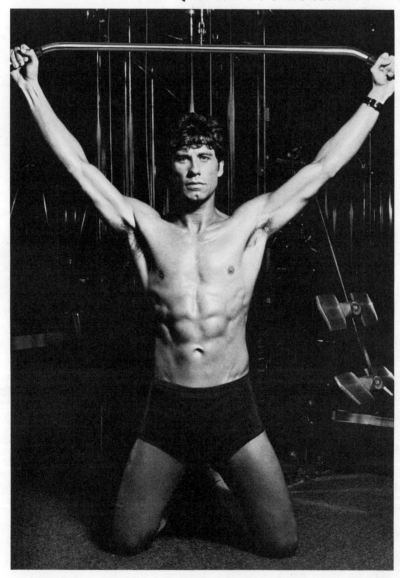

Begin by gripping the bar with hands as wide apart as possible while in a kneeling position. Pull the selected weight down as you kneel below the bar. Start with twenty or thirty pounds or a weight that you can comfortably pull for ten repetitions. The bar must be pulled down behind your head. If you find that your arms are not fully extended before the weight touches the stack, you will have to widen your knee stance.

Pull the bar down until it touches the back part of your neck. Slowly return the bar to the top and then immediately begin the next repetition. Concentrate on making your back work.

Exhale as you pull the bar down and inhale as the bar moves upward.

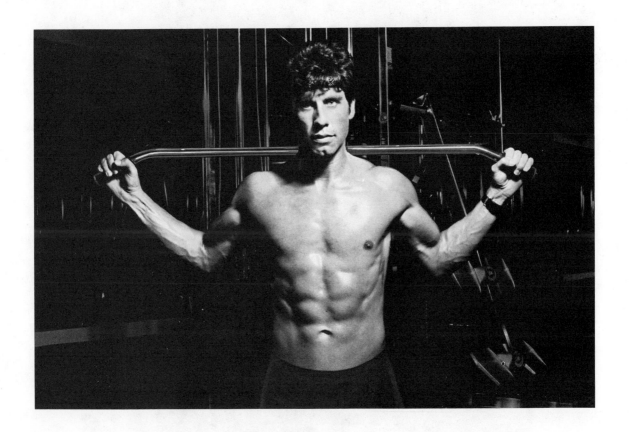

PULL-DOWNS (FRONT)

3 sets
10 repetitions

Pull-Downs in front work the lower part of your lats. This exercise will complete the work on this part of your back.

Position yourself correctly by making sure that when you pull down the cable will be in front of your nose. Grip the bar so your hands are about shoulder-width apart. Use twenty or thirty pounds for this exercise, or a weight that you can comfortably pull

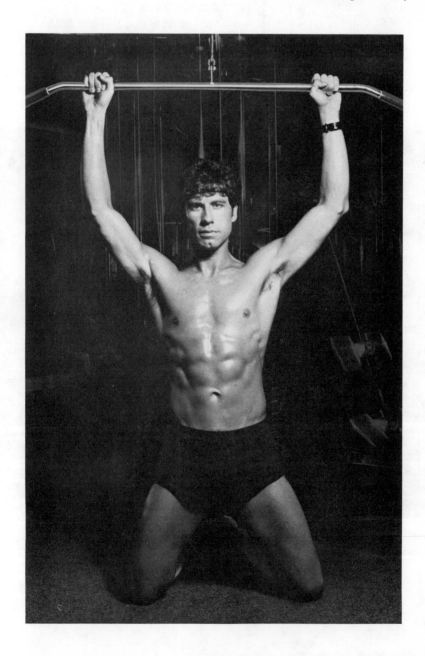

for ten repetitions. You will use a little less weight for this exercise than you used for the Pull-Downs in back.

Begin by pulling the bar down as you drop your elbows to your sides and lean back slightly. Pull the bar until it reaches your upper chest, then slowly return it to the starting position. Concentrate on letting your lower lats do the work.

Exhale as you pull the bar downward and inhale as you let the bar move upward to the starting position.

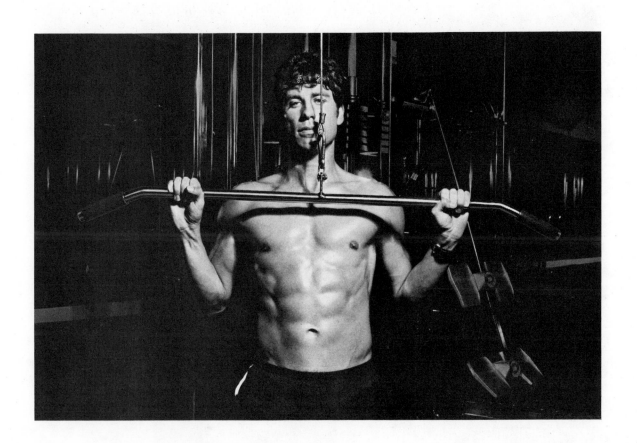

POSTURE LOW ROW

3 sets
10 repetitions

This is a great exercise for developing the lats and strengthening the lower back. Sit on the floor facing the low pulley with your legs extended and knees slightly bent. Grip the handles by bending forward at the waist. Your grip should be narrow, hands six to eight inches apart.

Begin by bending your elbows and pulling the handles toward your body, moving them slightly apart until they touch the area below your chest. Then slowly return to the starting position by extending your arms forward. Try not to move your upper body backward and forward during this movement.

Exhale as you pull the weight back and inhale as you return the weight to the starting position.

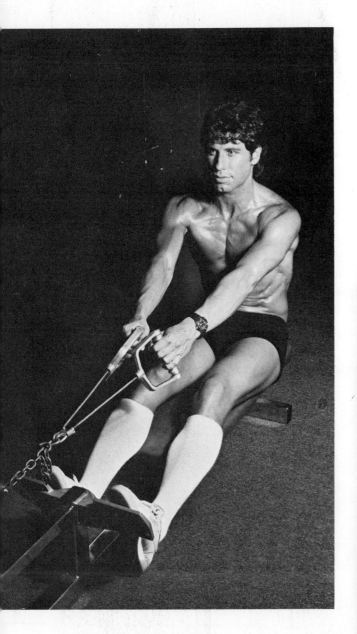

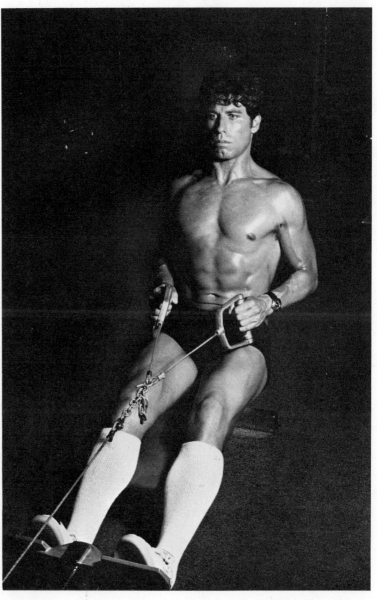

BARBELL DEAD LIFT

3 sets
10 repetitions

This is a great exercise for strengthening the lower back area, particularly the spinal erectors, the muscles that surround and support the lower spinal area.

Stand and hold the barbell with palms facing the body. Take a shoulder-width grip for this exercise. By bending at the waist let the barbell lower to about ankle level. If you cannot lower the barbell to your ankles then lower it as far as possible. Raise yourself back to the starting position by using the muscles of your lower back.

Inhale as you lower the weight and exhale as you return to the starting position.

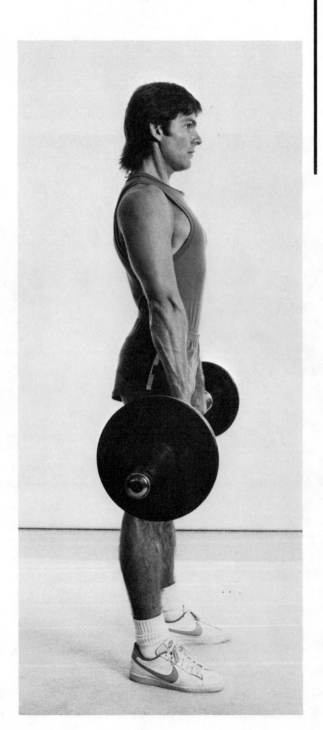

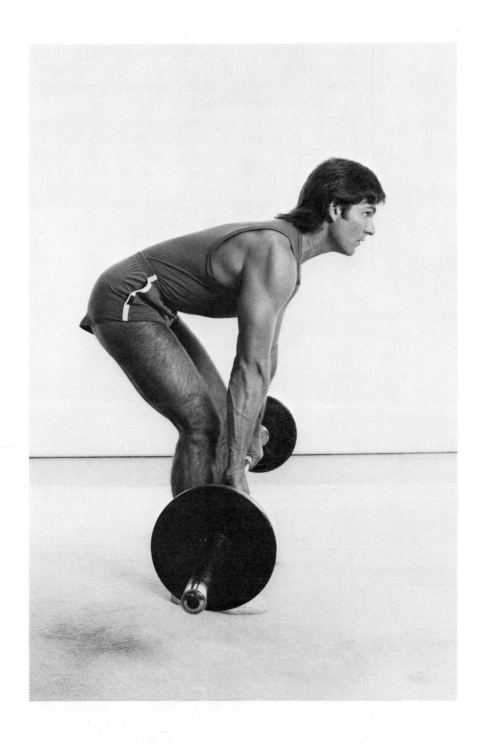

SHRUGS

3 sets
10 repetitions

The trapezius or upper back is often a neglected area. It is a very important muscle group that helps to keep the back straight.

Do this exercise by using the bench press. Back into the bench press and bend your knees before picking up the weight. Start with twenty or thirty pounds or a weight that you can comfortably lift for ten repetitions. Grip the handles in the middle, keeping your head up, back straight and knees bent. Pick up the weight and straighten your legs.

Begin by pushing your shoulders toward your ears. Shrug up as far as possible, hold for a count of one and then slowly lower your shoulders. Make sure you do not bend your elbows while doing the exercise.

Remember to bend your knees when putting the weight back down at the end of the exercise.

Exhale as you shrug shoulders toward ears and inhale as you lower them.

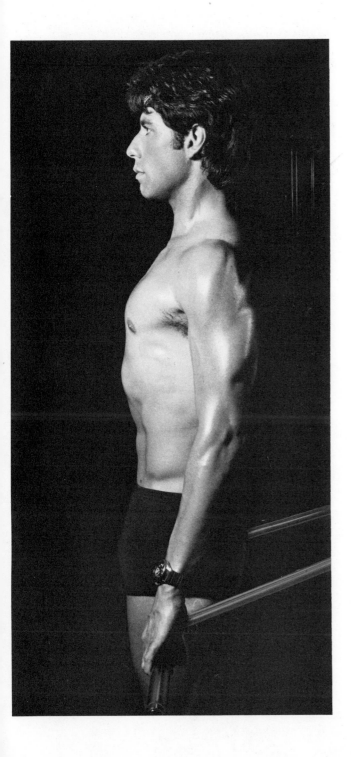 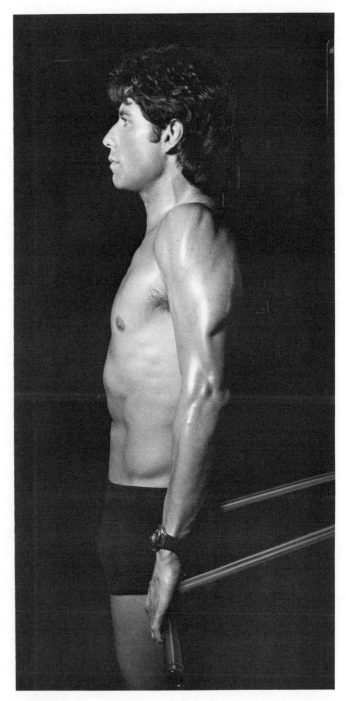

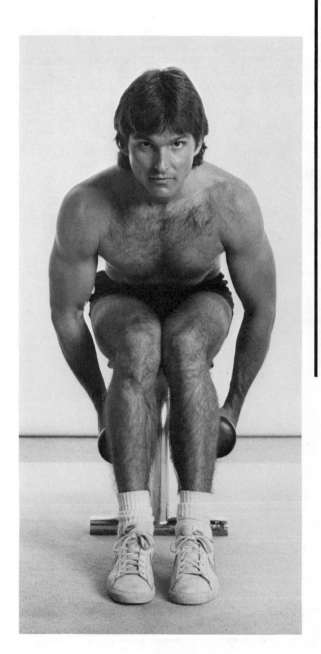

Shoulders and Arms

BENT LATERAL RAISES

3 sets
10 repetitions

Bent Lateral Raises strengthen the posterior deltoid muscles. This is the perfect exercise to do following your shrug work. It will help to develop a smooth tie-in between the trapezius and rear deltoid muscles. Use the flat bench for this exercise and start with the five- or ten-pound dumbbells or a weight you can comfortably raise for ten repetitions.

Sit on the end of the bench with feet about twelve inches in front of you. Grip the dumbbells so that your palms are facing each other beneath your upper legs. Bend over slightly until your lower stomach almost touches your thighs. Keep your back and head straight while in this position.

Begin by raising your arms until the dumbbells are level with your head. As your arms reach the top of the movement your back and head will rise slightly. Push your wrists upward slightly as you raise the weight. Lower the dumbbells slowly. Just before the dumbbells touch each other in the down position, begin the next repetition.

Exhale as you raise your arms and inhale as you lower them.

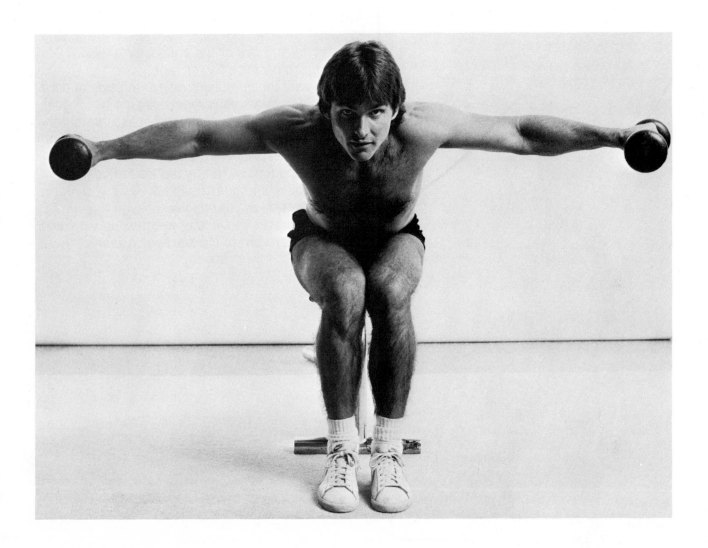

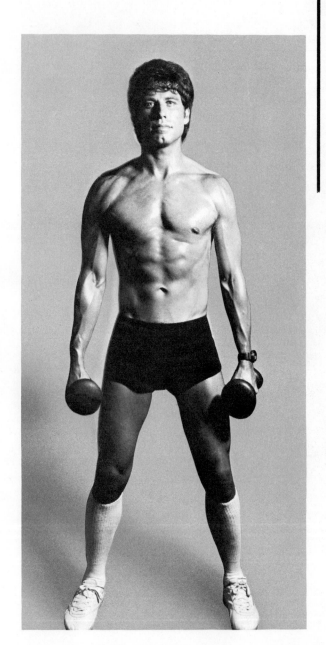

LATERAL RAISES

3 sets
10 repetitions

This exercise will strengthen the side deltoid or shoulder muscle. Do this exercise in a standing position holding five or ten pounds or a weight you can comfortably raise for ten repetitions.

Begin with the dumbbells held at the side of each leg. Slightly bend your legs, keeping your back straight and eyes forward. Slowly raise the dumbbells to shoulder level. Drop your hands slightly and push your wrists upward as you raise the dumbbells. This motion will further isolate the side deltoid muscle. Lower the dumbbells slowly as you return them to the side of your thighs.

Exhale as you move the weights upward and inhale as you return to the starting position.

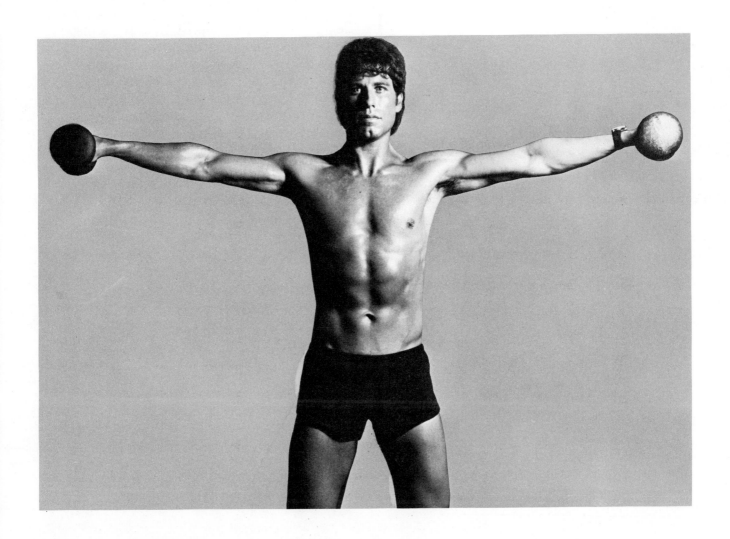

SHOULDER PRESS

3 sets
10 repetitions

The Shoulder Press is a great way to strengthen the anterior deltoid muscle. Use the shoulder press for this exercise. Start with twenty or thirty pounds, or a weight you can comfortably press for ten repetitions.

Begin by positioning the seat under the machine and sitting so your back is facing the weights. Move backward so your shoulders are even with the handles. With your back and head straight, secure your feet on the lower bars of the bench. Firmly grip the middle of each handle.

Push the weight upward and backward until your arms are fully extended. Then lower your arms by dropping your elbows. Continue as far as possible or until the weight touches the stack, then begin the next repetition.

Exhale as you press the weight upward and inhale as you lower the weight.

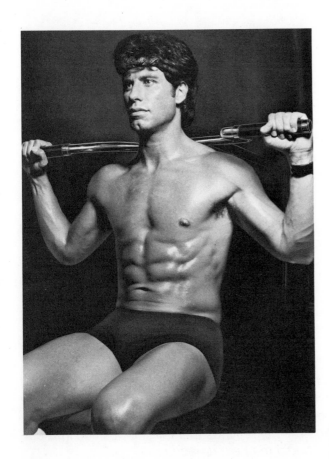

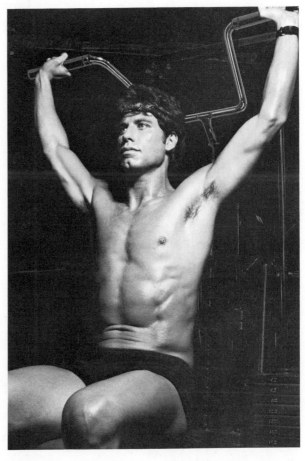

PRESS-DOWNS

2 sets
10 repetitions

The Press-Down is the best overall exercise for triceps development. You will use the same type of equipment that you used for the lat Pull-Downs (page 222). Start with twenty to thirty pounds, or a weight you can comfortably handle for ten repetitions.

Begin the exercise by gripping the bar in a standing position with hands about four inches apart, palms down. Keep your back, legs and head straight throughout the exercise. Feet should be shoulder-width apart. It is very important that you keep your elbows at your sides throughout the exercise. If you feel any pressure on your back move one foot slightly in front of the other.

Bring the bar down so it is even with the middle part of your chest. Begin the exercise by straightening the elbows and pushing the bar down until it touches your thighs. Hold in this position for a count of two, then slowly return to the starting position. When the bar reaches the starting position immediately begin the next repetition.

Exhale as you press the bar down and inhale as you let the bar up.

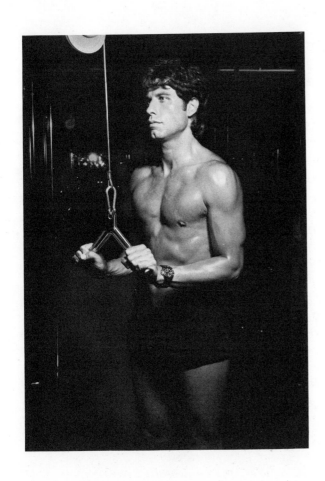

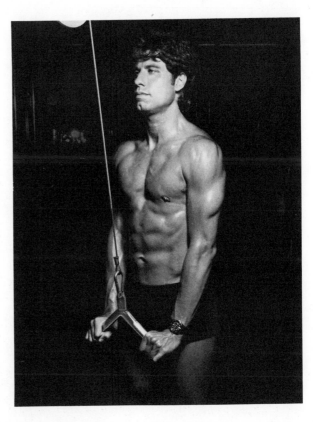

ONE-ARM EXTENSION

2 sets
10 repetitions each arm

The One-Arm Extension is a great exercise that works the triceps muscles. Sit on a flat bench holding a five- or ten-pound dumbbell behind your neck. Work up to heavier weights gradually. The palm of your hand should be facing the back of your neck. Your elbow should be close to the side of your head. Your opposite hand should be palm down next to your knee with your back straight and eyes forward.

Keeping your upper arm stationary, straighten your elbow and move the dumbbell upward until your arm is fully extended. Then slowly return to the starting position. Do ten repetitions with each arm.

Exhale as you push the weight upward and inhale as you lower the dumbbell.

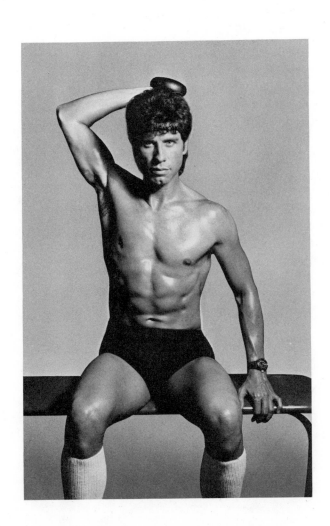

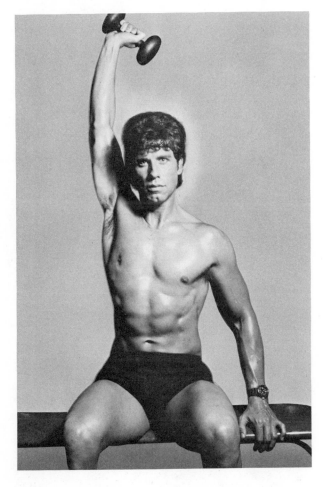

DIPS

2 sets
15 repetitions

Dips are a great way to finish your triceps workout. You will use the dip station for this.

Stand with your back to the dip station. Grip the ends of the handles in the palms-down position. Elbows should be back. Push yourself up to the starting position by fully extending your arms. In this position your chest should be tilted forward, slightly in front of your legs.

Begin by bending your elbows and lowering yourself until your forearms and upper arm touch. Your legs should be pushed behind you, bent, and your chest pushed forward. Push yourself back up by extending your arms. Then immediately begin the next repetition.

Inhale as you move down and exhale as you push up.

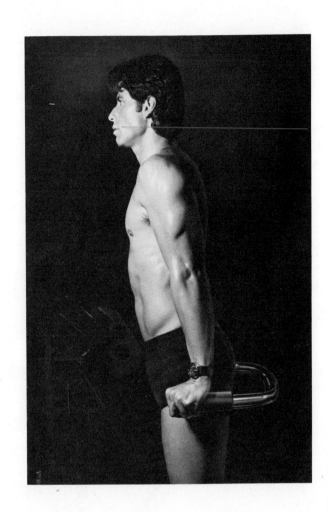

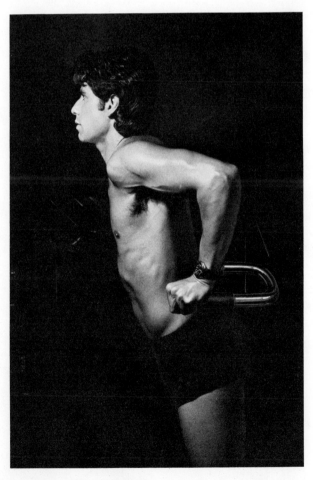

ALTERNATE SEATED CURLS

2 sets
10 repetitions, alternating arms

This is a great biceps exercise. It strengthens the entire biceps. Use a flat bench and the five- or ten-pound dumbbells, or a weight you can comfortably lift for ten repetitions.

Sit on the end of the bench with the dumbbells hanging at your sides. Grip the dumbbells firmly with palms facing the sides of the bench. Keep your back and head straight. Feet should be in front of you flat on the floor.

Begin with the right arm and turn your wrist so that your palm faces toward you as you begin to curl

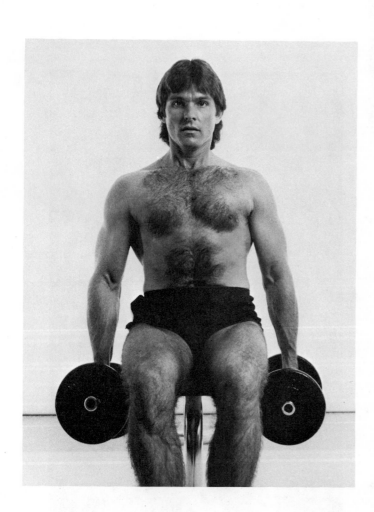

the dumbbell up. This means turning your right wrist clockwise. As you raise your forearm make sure your upper arm remains at your side. Squeeze your biceps at the top before lowering your arm. Just before your arm is fully lowered, turn your wrist to the starting position before beginning the next repetition with the other arm. Make sure you keep the dumbbell parallel with the floor as you raise and lower it.

Exhale as you curl the weight up and inhale as you lower the weight.

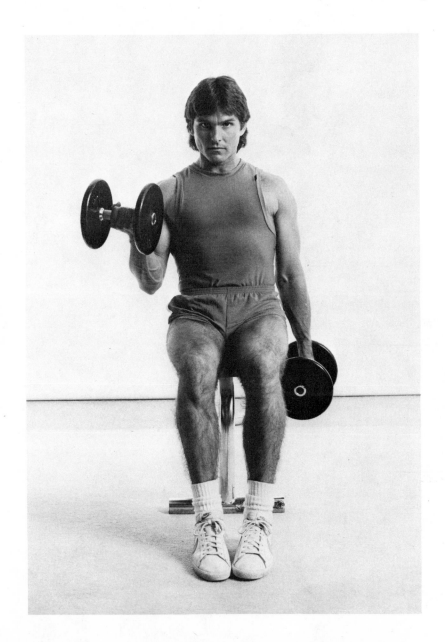

INCLINE CURLS

2 sets
10 repetitions

Incline Curls will work the upper biceps muscle. Use the incline bench for this exercise and the five- or ten-pound dumbbells, or a weight you can comfortably lift for ten repetitions.

Lie on the incline bench at a 45-degree angle. Dumbbells should be at your sides with arms hanging down and palms forward. Your back should be flat against the incline bench with your head slightly off the pad.

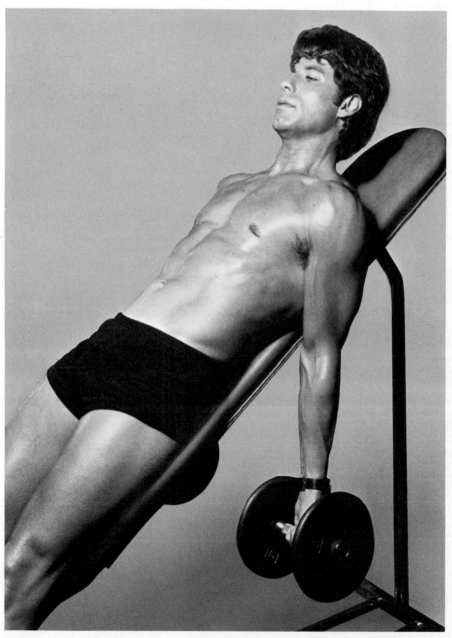

Begin by curling both dumbbells up, pulling your forearms toward your shoulders. Keep the upper arms stationary. Pull the dumbbells up until your forearms touch your biceps and then slowly lower the dumbbells, keeping them parallel to the floor at all times. Fully extend your arm at the bottom before beginning the next repetition.

Exhale as the weight is curled upward and inhale as you lower the weight.

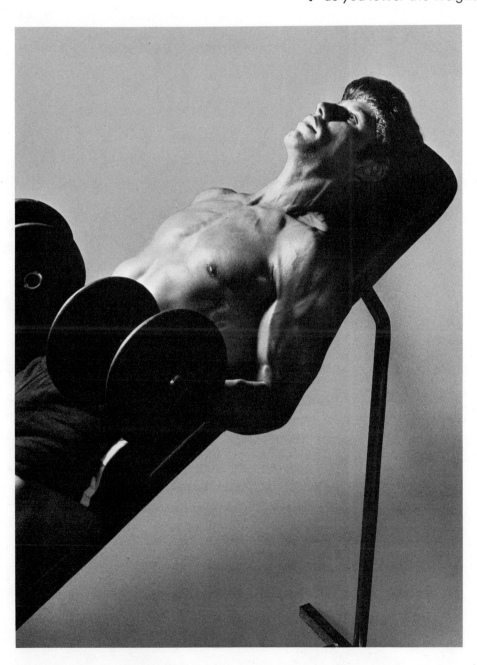

SEVENS

2 sets
21 repetitions

This is a perfect way to end your biceps workout. It is one of my favorite exercises. This exercise will work the entire biceps. Use the low pulley for this exercise. Start with ten or twenty pounds, or a weight that you can comfortably curl for at least ten repetitions.

Stand about twelve inches away from the low pulley station or far enough so that your arms are fully extended when the bar is in hand with palms up. Take a medium-width grip. Keep your back, legs and neck straight during this exercise, and your elbows at your sides. Do all three parts of the exercise without pause in between.

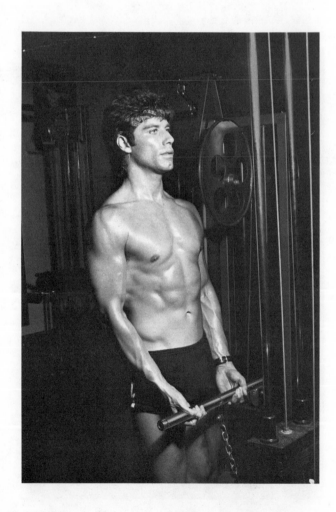

Begin by curling the bar up until your forearm is parallel with the floor, then return to the starting position. Do this seven times.

Then, starting with your forearms parallel to the floor immediately begin curling the weight to your shoulders, and then slowly return to the position with your forearms parallel to the floor. Do this seven times.

Finally lower the weight to the starting position with your arms straight and do a full set of seven complete curls to your shoulder.

Exhale as you curl the weight upward and inhale as you lower the weight.

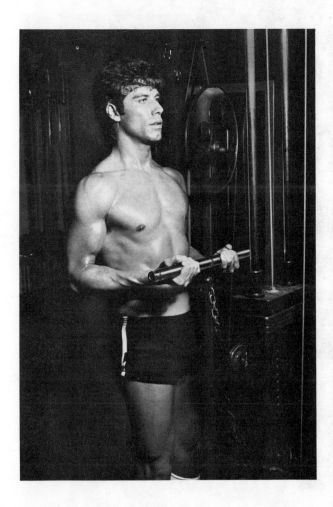
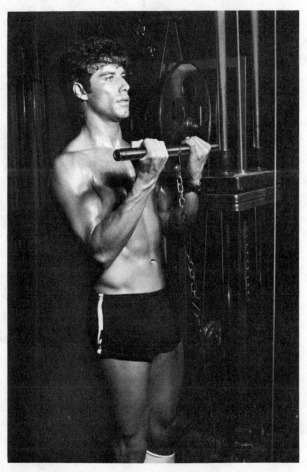

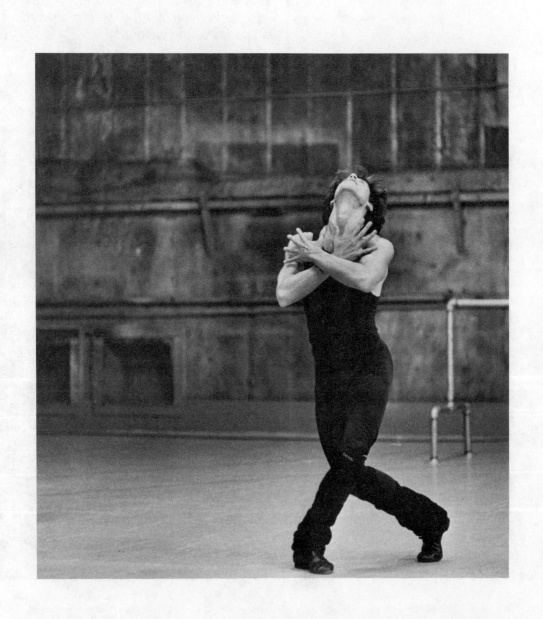

TIPS ON DIET AND HEALTH

Diet

Diet is such an individual thing, varying from person to person according to general background, food allergies, and overall health history, that I can't really make any formal recommendations in this area. All I can do is offer some general guidelines and tell you what I do.

First, I strongly suggest seeing a nutritionist or dietician of some sort. I use an M.D. who specializes in herbs, nutrition and natural remedies. This way I am supervised by someone who is a professional and highly trained.

During my training for *Staying Alive* I used a high-protein diet in combination with a vitamin program. It helped me to lose weight while keeping strong. Sometimes I found it hard to digest the vitamins. This is why I recommend an individual diet made by a doctor or nutritionist who can judge your individual body chemistry. Not everyone needs to lose weight. Perhaps you need to gain it, or perhaps you need an herbal regime instead of a vitamin program. Maybe you should eat certain foods and stay away from others. Whatever the case may be, having an individual diet prepared for you by an expert will give you more confidence in your program. Here are a few general suggestions that helped me:

1. Eat *fresh* fish, turkey, and chicken, and try to cut down on your consumption of red meat.
2. Eat fresh fruit and vegetables.
3. Drink eight to twelve 8-ounce glasses of water each day.

4. Eat fresh fruit in between meals if you are hungry.
5. Do not drink water or liquid with your meals other than to clear your mouth or throat if necessary.
6. Eat a salad with your meals. This will aid in the digestion process.
7. Restrict your use of salt, dairy products, and caffeine.
8. Do not eat any food past 6:00 P.M. Try to eat your last meal between 5:00 and 6:00 P.M.
9. Relax while eating and chew all your food throughly.
10. Do not drink extremely hot or cold liquids.

Nowadays there is considerable conversation regarding vitamins. Everyone wants to know how much and what type of vitamins are necessary and when to take them. During my training for *Staying Alive,* I chose a simple approach for my vitamin usage. I believe that proper eating will allow you to use vitamins as a *food supplement.*

I took a natural source of vitamins which includes a multivitamin and mineral formula, B complex, C and E. A good multivitamin formula with minerals is essential as a base for all your vitamin supplements. Extra B complex is important because it is not stored in the body. There are many factors which deprive foods and the body of needed B vitamins, such as stress, caffeine, alcohol and certain food-processing methods.

Vitamin C is also used up rapidly under stress and is excreted from the body in two to three hours. Therefore it is important to maintain a consistent level of vitamin C in your system.

Vitamin E is an antioxidant and helps to prevent fatigue. Like B and C, it is stored in the body for short periods of time.

Occasionally I would also use lipotropics to assist in burning fat, and digestive enzymes to aid my digestion. I used vitamin supplements at every lunch and dinner after finishing the meal. One day each week refrain from taking any vitamins at all.

The following was my vitamin program during *Staying Alive:*

Lunch
(1) Multivitamin and mineral tablet
(1) B complex
(1) C
(1) E

Dinner
(1) Multivitamin and mineral tablet
(1) C
(1) E

I didn't take extra vitamin B complex at dinner because it can make me restless and unable to sleep. Other than these daily supplements I took other vitamins or supplements only when I felt my body needed them. I think it is important to listen to your body and tune yourself into what you really need physically.

A lot of the credit for the new me goes to the change in my diet. Along with exercising, the food and vitamins you eat are an essential part of any plan to make yourself over.

Hair and Skin Care

When I was out of shape and not feeling good about myself physically, I started to notice I was losing a small amount of hair around my forehead and the top of my head. I began seeing a scalp treatment specialist, twice a week at first, then once a week. She gave me a scalp massage and a product treatment. These treatments seemed to stabilize the condition of both the hair and scalp.

Later that year I started my workout program in preparation for *Staying Alive,* and I noticed that the combination of the treatments and workouts made my hair even stronger. I'm sure the increased circulation of blood from working out improved the health of my scalp. Currently I'm experimenting with additional herbs and shampoo treatments. So far there seems to be even more improvement, and both my hair and scalp are in great shape.

Before this, at the same time that problems with my scalp occurred, I noticed that my skin seemed to be drier than usual, especially on my face. Later I learned that the condition of both my scalp and skin could have been due to lack of adequate circulation through lack of exercise. The workouts definitely helped correct these problems.

Anyway, I began to get facials on a weekly basis to cleanse my skin and keep it healthy. I am now experimenting with additional herbs, and with keeping the circulation going by working out. I have found that diet and exercise are the most important elements in keeping my hair, scalp, and skin in great shape.

Staying in Shape

Many people ask me how I keep the same physical condition I developed for *Staying Alive* now that I can no longer train six days a week. The key for me is diet. First, as I said earlier, once you're in shape it's much easier to stay that way. And second, being in good shape makes it much easier for me to control what I eat.

Even when not training for a specific role, I continue the same diet and nutritional program I use when in training. I may loosen the diet up a bit to include more variety, but essentially I keep the program the same.

To maintain my shape and size, I train with weights three days a week for about an hour each session using the Advanced format that I have given you in this book. I work all muscle groups, using two or three sets per exercise. I start with the warm-up dance routine, then move through all the other exercises, making sure my last several repetitions of each exercise are "completed to failure."

On a good week where I have some time to spare, I may take dance classes on the non-weight-lifting days. Sometimes I substitute another kind of aerobic exercise such as running, bicycling, or swimming. Be as creative as you like. Along with the proper diet, this kind of program keeps you in good condition. I stress diet because if you're careful about what you eat and behave fairly well, you will be able to work out as little as I do in this maintenance program.

This will not keep you in the kind of shape you would be in during heavy training, but I never seem to be more than a couple of weeks away from regaining this condition. So my maintenance program will keep you in a good place to work from, and it's a workable regime for everyday living.

The program in this book worked for me, and it changed my life. I want to share it with you.

Take care.